# POWER UP

SET GOALS, GET RESULTS

# POWER UP

# A WEIGHT LIFTER'S
# WORKOUT JOURNAL

Kalli Youngstrom

R
ROCKRIDGE
PRESS

Interior and Cover Designer: Heather Krakora

Art Producer: Hannah Dickerson

Editor: Natasha Yglesias

Production Editor: Mia Moran

GoGraph/serazetdinov and Can Stock Photo Inc./sangidan, cover and p. iii; iStock/ Designer, pp. i, viii, 1, 10, 11, 14, 15; Shutterstock/Lina_Lisichka, pp. 8-9

Author photo courtesy of Blair Knox Photography

ISBN: Print 978-1-64611-762-8

R0

# CONTENTS

# INTRODUCTION

Welcome to your new strength journal. I'm your coach,
Kalli Youngstrom!

This journal is a place to set goals, make promises to yourself, and
hold yourself accountable. Consistency is the key to success,
and accountability is the path to consistency. Make your commitment now. As Plato said, "Excellence is not a gift, but a skill that
takes practice."

Consider this not just an investment in your present self but an
investment in your physical retirement fund for future you. Consistent and dedicated weight training is one of the most affordable
forms of preventive medicine around, and its effects span from the
brain to the body—with benefits beyond what we see in the mirror
(and the personal records in this journal).

As a result of weight training, we're more likely to maintain a healthy
body composition through increased lean muscle mass and
decreased body fat (it's true, muscle burns more calories than fat);
and, we're also more likely to maintain a healthy mind due to an
increase in dopamine and other "feel good" hormones that work to
keep us happy and healthy. This can aid in reducing anxiousness
and sadness and even help combat the development of neurologi-
cal disorders such as Alzheimer's disease in the long term.

Consistent weight training prevents bone density loss and aids
in bone development, greatly decreasing the risk of osteoporo-
sis and helping lower the risk of resulting fractures. Along with
strengthening muscles and bones, weight training aids in strengthening joints, tendons, and ligaments, too. This allows us to maintain
strength and a better quality of life by lowering the risks of joint
pain and arthritis.

We want to be happy, healthy, and strong—not just for now but
for the future.

# HOW TO USE THIS BOOK

This journal is color coded so you can easily access different tools and sections. Part 1 is designed to set you up for success moving forward, with a variety of tips and tools to make the most of training and optimize progress. From body analysis to exercise options to goal setting, part 1 is a resource to reference time and again throughout any training program. It will serve as a reminder of where you started and where you want to go.

After setting goals and initial assessments, you can begin your fitness journey with a focused mind prepared for progress. Part 2 allows space for recording progress in both strength and body composition in order to ensure that you're on track to achieve the goals you've set for yourself.

Part 3 is where you'll find yourself on a more daily basis. This section provides space to track daily workouts and the details surrounding them, including energy, mood, and meals, in order to optimize the many variables that impact the quality of workouts and recovery.

# PART ONE

# START STRONG

## GET STARTED

The difference between a dream and a goal is a plan, and this journal is a part of your plan. As you move forward with clear goal setting and daily tracking, you'll be holding yourself accountable and setting yourself up for success. As Epictetus said, "First tell yourself what kind of person you want to be, then do what you have to do." As you turn the pages of this journal, it's a reflection of you putting your future in your own hands, a commitment to becoming the person you want to be. Congratulations on taking the first step!

# SUCCESS TIPS

When it comes to successfully achieving strength goals and progressing in training, it's just as important to focus on what you're doing outside the gym as it is to focus on what you're doing in it. Take care of yourself with proper nutrition, hydration, rest, and recovery in order to stay healthy and injury-free.

## water

» Aim for 3 to 4 liters of water a day. Our bodies like consistency, so try to keep a regular daily intake (and, no, coffee doesn't count).

» If supplements are in the budget, a branched-chain amino acid (BCAA) is a great addition to your $H_2O$. It will help with muscle development and recovery.

## nutrition

» Ensure that you're achieving adequate calorie and protein intake to support training and recovery.

» You can't outtrain a bad diet. Food is fuel! Be conscious of what you're putting in your body.

## rest & recovery

» Along with planning training days, prioritize rest days as well. Bodies need time to recover, so take a minimum of one day off weekly for active rest.

» Stretching, foam rolling, massage, and yoga all assist in recovery. Try these and see what works best for you.

» Sleep is one of the most underrated variables when it comes to strength progression. Aim for seven to eight hours of sleep a night.

» Poor sleep or lack of sleep leads to increased cortisol, greater injury risk, and delayed recovery.

Prioritize goal setting and planning in these areas, along with your training. Keep track of your food and water intake, schedule rest days and recovery activities, and create a regular sleep schedule and hold yourself accountable to it. Not only will these aid in the progression of strength and training, but they'll also help keep you happy, healthy, and balanced from the inside out. You'll be running like a well-oiled machine!

# BODY STATS

There are many ways to measure progress and assess change when it comes to health and fitness. I recommend performing several different assessments in order to gain a complete picture. Remember, the scale isn't the only indicator of success, and quite often it can be deceiving. As you move forward within a training program, you may notice the number on the scale increase, fluctuate, or plateau, all of which can be discouraging depending on your goals.

The number on the scale can be impacted by many variables. Due to the variance that occurs, one of my preferred assessment methods is body composition or body fat percentage. It's a great indicator of general health and a more accurate representation of true physical progress.

There are several different approaches to measuring body fat percentage, and they vary in both accuracy and accessibility. The most common are calipers and handheld devices, or bioelectrical impedance analysis (BIA), which many gyms and trainers use. Although these options may not be the most accurate, they're the most accurate of the more accessible testing methods.

Other analyses that may be more accurate but are more difficult to access for most include things like Bod Pods, DXA Scans, and hydrostatic weighing. For our purposes, we'll focus on the most frequently used approach, which is skinfold calipers. Use the following chart to assess and update your body as it changes moving forward. For more information, you can visit MuscleAndStrength.com, go to the tools section, and then go to the body fat percentage calculator.

# CALIPER MEASURES

| DATE | | | | |
|---|---|---|---|---|
| BODY WEIGHT | | | | |
| BODY AREA | MEASUREMENT | MEASUREMENT | MEASUREMENT | MEASUREMENT |
| | | | | |
| | | | | |
| | | | | |
| | | | | |
| | | | | |
| | | | | |
| Caliper Subtotals | | | | |
| Body Fat % | | | | |
| Lean Body Mass | | | | |

# SET YOUR GOALS

To support successful goal setting, I use the SMART acronym. This stands for specific, measurable, achievable, realistic, and timebound. It's easy to reach for the stars when setting goals, and you should, but it's also important to set yourself up for success. This means setting a realistic, specific goal—one that can be measured— and one with a deadline. For example: Setting a specific deadlift personal record (PR) goal by the time you reach the end of this journal is specific, measurable, achievable, realistic, and timebound. I also recommend setting goals focused on a variety of markers related to well-being, such as health, function, fitness, and physique. This decreases the likelihood of becoming hyperfocused on one thing (such as the scale) and ignoring the rest.

For example:

**HEALTH GOAL:** lowering blood sugar/blood pressure; increasing or decreasing body fat as necessary

**FITNESS GOAL:** running a 10K for a new PR; achieving your first bodyweight pull-up

**FUNCTION GOAL:** comfortably hiking on holiday pain free; maintaining strength for lifting at work

**PHYSIQUE GOAL:** feeling confident and fitting comfortably into your favorite jeans

Date: _____

My Goals: _____

_____

_____

_____

_____

# MAKE IT MEASURABLE

Here, you can track current and future assessments for both body and strength measurements. If you don't have goal measurements, you can use this column for your final measurements instead. Use a flexible-fabric measuring tape and measure the circumference of each body part at its largest point.

| DATE | | |
|---|---|---|
| **BODY MEASUREMENTS** | **CURRENT** | **GOAL** |
| Body Weight | | |
| Body Fat % | | |
| Upper Arms | | |
| Chest | | |
| Waist | | |
| Hips | | |
| Thighs | | |
| Calves | | |
| Other: _____ | | |
| **STRENGTH MEASUREMENTS** | | |
| Bench Press | | |
| Barbell Squat | | |
| Barbell Deadlift | | |
| Bent-Overhead Press | | |
| Snatch | | |
| Clean & Jerk | | |
| Lat Raise | | |
| Bent-Over Row | | |
| Bicep Curl | | |
| Tricep Extension | | |
| Other: _____ | | |
| Other: _____ | | |

# ANATOMY TUTORIAL

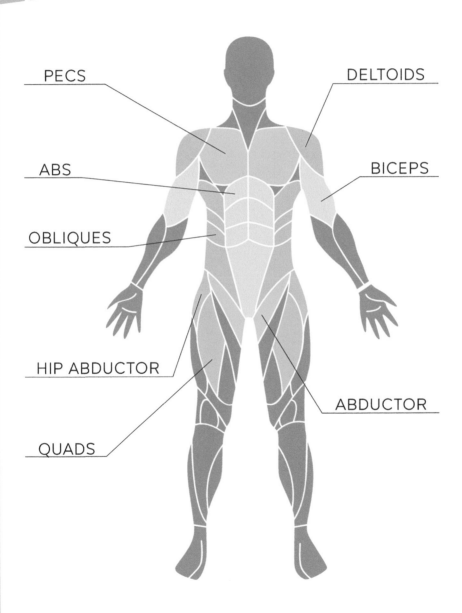

PECS

DELTOIDS

ABS

BICEPS

OBLIQUES

HIP ABDUCTOR

ABDUCTOR

QUADS

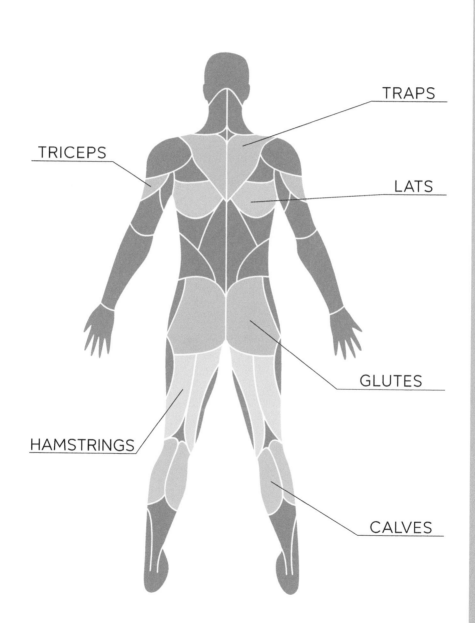

TRAPS

TRICEPS

LATS

GLUTES

HAMSTRINGS

CALVES

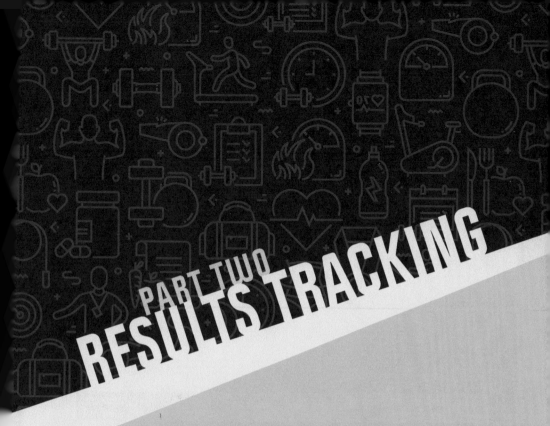

# PART TWO

# RESULTS TRACKING

## RESULTS LOG

The logs are a dedicated space to track your physical and strength assessments monthly or as you see fit. I recommend at least monthly, but this may vary depending on your goals. I find that a monthly review and re-assessment is the perfect way to stay focused on the health, fitness, function, and physique goals I've laid out for myself and to ensure that I'm on track. Remember that measurements are based on circumference. (See part 1's "Make It Measurable" for details.)

|  | **DATE** | | | | | |
|---|---|---|---|---|---|---|
| **BODY MEASUREMENTS** | | | | | | |
| Body Weight | | | | | | |
| Body Fat % | | | | | | |
| Upper Arms | | | | | | |
| Chest | | | | | | |
| Waist | | | | | | |
| Hips | | | | | | |
| Thighs | | | | | | |
| Calves | | | | | | |
| Other: _____ | | | | | | |
| **STRENGTH MEASUREMENTS** | | | | | | |
| Snatch | | | | | | |
| Barbell Squat | | | | | | |
| Bent-Over Row | | | | | | |
| Bench Press | | | | | | |
| Deadlift | | | | | | |
| Lat Raise | | | | | | |
| Barbell Curl | | | | | | |
| Tricep Press | | | | | | |
| Other: _____ | | | | | | |
| Other: _____ | | | | | | |
| Other: _____ | | | | | | |

| DATE | | | | | |
|---|---|---|---|---|---|
| **BODY MEASUREMENTS** | | | | | |
| Body Weight | | | | | |
| Body Fat % | | | | | |
| Upper Arms | | | | | |
| Chest | | | | | |
| Waist | | | | | |
| Hips | | | | | |
| Thighs | | | | | |
| Calves | | | | | |
| Other: _____ | | | | | |
| **STRENGTH MEASUREMENTS** | | | | | |
| Snatch | | | | | |
| Barbell Squat | | | | | |
| Bent-Over Row | | | | | |
| Bench Press | | | | | |
| Deadlift | | | | | |
| Lat Raise | | | | | |
| Barbell Curl | | | | | |
| Tricep Press | | | | | |
| Other: _____ | | | | | |
| Other: _____ | | | | | |
| Other: _____ | | | | | |

# PART THREE

# WORKOUT LOGS

## TRACK YOUR WORKOUT

Welcome to your daily space for personal check-ins. This not only is for tracking workouts but also details surrounding workouts that may impact performance and recovery. I consider this not just an accountability check-in but a time to check in with your body and mind to ensure that you're optimizing both physical and mental health. Take note of any patterns that may occur.

Date: _____

Day of the Week: S ☐   M ☐   T ☐   W ☐   R ☐   F ☐   S ☐

Start Time: _____   Finish Time: _____

Stretch/Warm-Up: Yes ☐   No ☐

Cardio: _____   Level: _____

Pre-Workout Mood and Energy: _____

Pre-Workout Food/Snack: _____

## MUSCLE GROUP EMPHASIZED

Chest ☐   Shoulders ☐   Back ☐   Arms ☐
Legs ☐   Abs ☐   None ☐

## WORKOUT QUALITY

Low ☐   Okay ☐   Good ☐   Great ☐

Post-Workout Mood and Energy: _____

_____

Post-Workout Food/Snack: _____

_____

_____

Notes: _____

_____

_____

_____

_____

_____

| MUSCLE GROUP | SET 1 | | SET 2 | | SET 3 | | SET 4 | | SET 5 | |
|---|---|---|---|---|---|---|---|---|---|---|
| EXERCISE | REPS | WGT | REPS | WGT | REPS | WGT | REPS | WGT | REPS | WGT |
| | | | | | | | | | | |
| | | | | | | | | | | |
| | | | | | | | | | | |
| | | | | | | | | | | |
| | | | | | | | | | | |
| | | | | | | | | | | |
| | | | | | | | | | | |
| | | | | | | | | | | |
| | | | | | | | | | | |
| | | | | | | | | | | |
| | | | | | | | | | | |
| | | | | | | | | | | |

Date: _____

Day of the Week:  S ☐    M ☐    T ☐    W ☐    R ☐    F ☐    S ☐

Start Time: _____    Finish Time: _____

Stretch/Warm-Up:  Yes ☐    No ☐

Cardio: _____    Level: _____

Pre-Workout Mood and Energy: _____

Pre-Workout Food/Snack: _____

## MUSCLE GROUP EMPHASIZED

Chest ☐    Shoulders ☐    Back ☐    Arms ☐
Legs ☐    Abs ☐    None ☐

## WORKOUT QUALITY

Low ☐    Okay ☐    Good ☐    Great ☐

Post-Workout Mood and Energy: _____

_____

Post-Workout Food/Snack: _____

_____

_____

Notes: _____

_____

_____

_____

_____

_____

| MUSCLE GROUP | SET 1 | | SET 2 | | SET 3 | | SET 4 | | SET 5 | |
|---|---|---|---|---|---|---|---|---|---|---|
| EXERCISE | REPS | WGT | REPS | WGT | REPS | WGT | REPS | WGT | REPS | WGT |
| | | | | | | | | | | |
| | | | | | | | | | | |
| | | | | | | | | | | |
| | | | | | | | | | | |
| | | | | | | | | | | |
| | | | | | | | | | | |
| | | | | | | | | | | |
| | | | | | | | | | | |
| | | | | | | | | | | |
| | | | | | | | | | | |
| | | | | | | | | | | |
| | | | | | | | | | | |

Date: _____

Day of the Week: S ☐    M ☐    T ☐    W ☐    R ☐    F ☐    S ☐

Start Time: _____    Finish Time: _____

Stretch/Warm-Up: Yes ☐    No ☐

Cardio: _____    Level: _____

Pre-Workout Mood and Energy: _____

Pre-Workout Food/Snack: _____

## MUSCLE GROUP EMPHASIZED

Chest ☐    Shoulders ☐    Back ☐    Arms ☐
Legs ☐    Abs ☐    None ☐

## WORKOUT QUALITY

Low ☐    Okay ☐    Good ☐    Great ☐

Post-Workout Mood and Energy: _____

_____

_____

Post-Workout Food/Snack: _____

_____

_____

Notes: _____

_____

_____

_____

_____

_____

_____

| MUSCLE GROUP | SET 1 | | SET 2 | | SET 3 | | SET 4 | | SET 5 | |
|---|---|---|---|---|---|---|---|---|---|---|
| EXERCISE | REPS | WGT | REPS | WGT | REPS | WGT | REPS | WGT | REPS | WGT |
| | | | | | | | | | | |
| | | | | | | | | | | |
| | | | | | | | | | | |
| | | | | | | | | | | |
| | | | | | | | | | | |
| | | | | | | | | | | |
| | | | | | | | | | | |
| | | | | | | | | | | |
| | | | | | | | | | | |
| | | | | | | | | | | |
| | | | | | | | | | | |

Date: _____

Day of the Week: S ☐   M ☐   T ☐   W ☐   R ☐   F ☐   S ☐

Start Time: _____   Finish Time: _____

Stretch/Warm-Up: Yes ☐   No ☐

Cardio: _____   Level: _____

Pre-Workout Mood and Energy: _____

Pre-Workout Food/Snack: _____

## MUSCLE GROUP EMPHASIZED

Chest ☐   Shoulders ☐   Back ☐   Arms ☐
Legs ☐   Abs ☐   None ☐

## WORKOUT QUALITY

Low ☐   Okay ☐   Good ☐   Great ☐

Post-Workout Mood and Energy: _____

_____

Post-Workout Food/Snack: _____

_____

_____

Notes: _____

_____

_____

_____

_____

_____

| MUSCLE GROUP | SET 1 | | SET 2 | | SET 3 | | SET 4 | | SET 5 | |
|---|---|---|---|---|---|---|---|---|---|---|
| EXERCISE | REPS | WGT | REPS | WGT | REPS | WGT | REPS | WGT | REPS | WGT |
| | | | | | | | | | | |
| | | | | | | | | | | |
| | | | | | | | | | | |
| | | | | | | | | | | |
| | | | | | | | | | | |
| | | | | | | | | | | |
| | | | | | | | | | | |
| | | | | | | | | | | |
| | | | | | | | | | | |
| | | | | | | | | | | |
| | | | | | | | | | | |

Date: _____

Day of the Week:  S ☐    M ☐    T ☐    W ☐    R ☐    F ☐    S ☐

Start Time: _____    Finish Time: _____

Stretch/Warm-Up:  Yes ☐    No ☐

Cardio: _____    Level: _____

Pre-Workout Mood and Energy: _____

Pre-Workout Food/Snack: _____

## MUSCLE GROUP EMPHASIZED

Chest ☐    Shoulders ☐    Back ☐    Arms ☐
Legs ☐    Abs ☐    None ☐

## WORKOUT QUALITY

Low ☐    Okay ☐    Good ☐    Great ☐

Post-Workout Mood and Energy: _____

_____

Post-Workout Food/Snack: _____

_____

_____

Notes: _____

_____

_____

_____

_____

_____

| MUSCLE GROUP | SET 1 | | SET 2 | | SET 3 | | SET 4 | | SET 5 | |
|---|---|---|---|---|---|---|---|---|---|---|
| **EXERCISE** | **REPS** | **WGT** | **REPS** | **WGT** | **REPS** | **WGT** | **REPS** | **WGT** | **REPS** | **WGT** |
| | | | | | | | | | | |
| | | | | | | | | | | |
| | | | | | | | | | | |
| | | | | | | | | | | |
| | | | | | | | | | | |
| | | | | | | | | | | |
| | | | | | | | | | | |
| | | | | | | | | | | |
| | | | | | | | | | | |
| | | | | | | | | | | |
| | | | | | | | | | | |

Date: _____

Day of the Week:  S ☐     M ☐     T ☐     W ☐     R ☐     F ☐     S ☐

Start Time: _____     Finish Time: _____

Stretch/Warm-Up:  Yes ☐     No ☐

Cardio: _____     Level: _____

Pre-Workout Mood and Energy: _____

Pre-Workout Food/Snack: _____

## MUSCLE GROUP EMPHASIZED

Chest ☐     Shoulders ☐     Back ☐     Arms ☐
Legs ☐     Abs ☐     None ☐

## WORKOUT QUALITY

Low ☐     Okay ☐     Good ☐     Great ☐

Post-Workout Mood and Energy: _____

_____

Post-Workout Food/Snack: _____

_____

_____

Notes: _____

_____

_____

_____

_____

_____

| MUSCLE GROUP | SET 1 | | SET 2 | | SET 3 | | SET 4 | | SET 5 | |
|---|---|---|---|---|---|---|---|---|---|---|
| EXERCISE | REPS | WGT | REPS | WGT | REPS | WGT | REPS | WGT | REPS | WGT |
| | | | | | | | | | | |
| | | | | | | | | | | |
| | | | | | | | | | | |
| | | | | | | | | | | |
| | | | | | | | | | | |
| | | | | | | | | | | |
| | | | | | | | | | | |
| | | | | | | | | | | |
| | | | | | | | | | | |
| | | | | | | | | | | |
| | | | | | | | | | | |
| | | | | | | | | | | |

Date: _____

Day of the Week:  S ☐   M ☐   T ☐   W ☐   R ☐   F ☐   S ☐

Start Time: _____   Finish Time: _____

Stretch/Warm-Up:  Yes ☐   No ☐

Cardio: _____   Level: _____

Pre-Workout Mood and Energy: _____

Pre-Workout Food/Snack: _____

## MUSCLE GROUP EMPHASIZED

Chest ☐   Shoulders ☐   Back ☐   Arms ☐
Legs ☐   Abs ☐   None ☐

## WORKOUT QUALITY

Low ☐   Okay ☐   Good ☐   Great ☐

Post-Workout Mood and Energy: _____

_____

Post-Workout Food/Snack: _____

_____

_____

Notes: _____

_____

_____

_____

_____

| MUSCLE GROUP | SET 1 | | SET 2 | | SET 3 | | SET 4 | | SET 5 | |
|---|---|---|---|---|---|---|---|---|---|---|
| EXERCISE | REPS | WGT | REPS | WGT | REPS | WGT | REPS | WGT | REPS | WGT |
| | | | | | | | | | | |
| | | | | | | | | | | |
| | | | | | | | | | | |
| | | | | | | | | | | |
| | | | | | | | | | | |
| | | | | | | | | | | |
| | | | | | | | | | | |
| | | | | | | | | | | |
| | | | | | | | | | | |
| | | | | | | | | | | |
| | | | | | | | | | | |

Date: _____

Day of the Week:  S ☐    M ☐    T ☐    W ☐    R ☐    F ☐    S ☐

Start Time: _____    Finish Time: _____

Stretch/Warm-Up:  Yes ☐    No ☐

Cardio: _____    Level: _____

Pre-Workout Mood and Energy: _____

Pre-Workout Food/Snack: _____

## MUSCLE GROUP EMPHASIZED

Chest ☐    Shoulders ☐    Back ☐    Arms ☐
Legs ☐    Abs ☐    None ☐

## WORKOUT QUALITY

Low ☐    Okay ☐    Good ☐    Great ☐

Post-Workout Mood and Energy: _____

_____

Post-Workout Food/Snack: _____

_____

_____

Notes: _____

_____

_____

_____

_____

_____

| MUSCLE GROUP | SET 1 | | SET 2 | | SET 3 | | SET 4 | | SET 5 | |
|---|---|---|---|---|---|---|---|---|---|---|
| EXERCISE | REPS | WGT | REPS | WGT | REPS | WGT | REPS | WGT | REPS | WGT |
| | | | | | | | | | | |
| | | | | | | | | | | |
| | | | | | | | | | | |
| | | | | | | | | | | |
| | | | | | | | | | | |
| | | | | | | | | | | |
| | | | | | | | | | | |
| | | | | | | | | | | |
| | | | | | | | | | | |
| | | | | | | | | | | |
| | | | | | | | | | | |

Date: _____

Day of the Week:  S ☐    M ☐    T ☐    W ☐    R ☐    F ☐    S ☐

Start Time: _____    Finish Time: _____

Stretch/Warm-Up: Yes ☐    No ☐

Cardio: _____    Level: _____

Pre-Workout Mood and Energy: _____

Pre-Workout Food/Snack: _____

## MUSCLE GROUP EMPHASIZED

Chest ☐    Shoulders ☐    Back ☐    Arms ☐
Legs ☐    Abs ☐    None ☐

## WORKOUT QUALITY

Low ☐    Okay ☐    Good ☐    Great ☐

Post-Workout Mood and Energy: _____

_____

Post-Workout Food/Snack: _____

_____

_____

Notes: _____

_____

_____

_____

_____

_____

| MUSCLE GROUP | SET 1 | | SET 2 | | SET 3 | | SET 4 | | SET 5 | |
|---|---|---|---|---|---|---|---|---|---|---|
| EXERCISE | REPS | WGT | REPS | WGT | REPS | WGT | REPS | WGT | REPS | WGT |
| | | | | | | | | | | |
| | | | | | | | | | | |
| | | | | | | | | | | |
| | | | | | | | | | | |
| | | | | | | | | | | |
| | | | | | | | | | | |
| | | | | | | | | | | |
| | | | | | | | | | | |
| | | | | | | | | | | |
| | | | | | | | | | | |

Date: _____

Day of the Week:  S ☐    M ☐    T ☐    W ☐    R ☐    F ☐    S ☐

Start Time: _____    Finish Time: _____

Stretch/Warm-Up:  Yes ☐    No ☐

Cardio: _____    Level: _____

Pre-Workout Mood and Energy: _____

Pre-Workout Food/Snack: _____

## MUSCLE GROUP EMPHASIZED

Chest ☐    Shoulders ☐    Back ☐    Arms ☐
Legs ☐    Abs ☐    None ☐

## WORKOUT QUALITY

Low ☐    Okay ☐    Good ☐    Great ☐

Post-Workout Mood and Energy: _____

_____

Post-Workout Food/Snack: _____

_____

_____

Notes: _____

_____

_____

_____

_____

_____

| MUSCLE GROUP | SET 1 | | SET 2 | | SET 3 | | SET 4 | | SET 5 | |
|---|---|---|---|---|---|---|---|---|---|---|
| EXERCISE | REPS | WGT | REPS | WGT | REPS | WGT | REPS | WGT | REPS | WGT |
| | | | | | | | | | | |
| | | | | | | | | | | |
| | | | | | | | | | | |
| | | | | | | | | | | |
| | | | | | | | | | | |
| | | | | | | | | | | |
| | | | | | | | | | | |
| | | | | | | | | | | |
| | | | | | | | | | | |
| | | | | | | | | | | |
| | | | | | | | | | | |
| | | | | | | | | | | |

Date: _____

Day of the Week:  S ☐    M ☐    T ☐    W ☐    R ☐    F ☐    S ☐

Start Time: _____    Finish Time: _____

Stretch/Warm-Up:  Yes ☐    No ☐

Cardio: _____    Level: _____

Pre-Workout Mood and Energy: _____

Pre-Workout Food/Snack: _____

## MUSCLE GROUP EMPHASIZED

Chest ☐    Shoulders ☐    Back ☐    Arms ☐
Legs ☐    Abs ☐    None ☐

## WORKOUT QUALITY

Low ☐    Okay ☐    Good ☐    Great ☐

Post-Workout Mood and Energy: _____

_____

Post-Workout Food/Snack: _____

_____

_____

Notes: _____

_____

_____

_____

_____

_____

| MUSCLE GROUP | SET 1 | | SET 2 | | SET 3 | | SET 4 | | SET 5 | |
|---|---|---|---|---|---|---|---|---|---|---|
| EXERCISE | REPS | WGT | REPS | WGT | REPS | WGT | REPS | WGT | REPS | WGT |
| | | | | | | | | | | |
| | | | | | | | | | | |
| | | | | | | | | | | |
| | | | | | | | | | | |
| | | | | | | | | | | |
| | | | | | | | | | | |
| | | | | | | | | | | |
| | | | | | | | | | | |
| | | | | | | | | | | |
| | | | | | | | | | | |
| | | | | | | | | | | |
| | | | | | | | | | | |

Date: _____

Day of the Week: S ☐    M ☐    T ☐    W ☐    R ☐    F ☐    S ☐

Start Time: _____    Finish Time: _____

Stretch/Warm-Up: Yes ☐    No ☐

Cardio: _____    Level: _____

Pre-Workout Mood and Energy: _____

Pre-Workout Food/Snack: _____

## MUSCLE GROUP EMPHASIZED

Chest ☐    Shoulders ☐    Back ☐    Arms ☐
Legs ☐    Abs ☐    None ☐

## WORKOUT QUALITY

Low ☐    Okay ☐    Good ☐    Great ☐

Post-Workout Mood and Energy: _____

_____

Post-Workout Food/Snack: _____

_____

_____

Notes: _____

_____

_____

_____

_____

_____

| MUSCLE GROUP | SET 1 | | SET 2 | | SET 3 | | SET 4 | | SET 5 | |
|---|---|---|---|---|---|---|---|---|---|---|
| EXERCISE | REPS | WGT | REPS | WGT | REPS | WGT | REPS | WGT | REPS | WGT |
| | | | | | | | | | | |
| | | | | | | | | | | |
| | | | | | | | | | | |
| | | | | | | | | | | |
| | | | | | | | | | | |
| | | | | | | | | | | |
| | | | | | | | | | | |
| | | | | | | | | | | |
| | | | | | | | | | | |
| | | | | | | | | | | |
| | | | | | | | | | | |

Date: _____

Day of the Week:  S ☐   M ☐   T ☐   W ☐   R ☐   F ☐   S ☐

Start Time: _____   Finish Time: _____

Stretch/Warm-Up:  Yes ☐    No ☐

Cardio: _____   Level: _____

Pre-Workout Mood and Energy: _____

Pre-Workout Food/Snack: _____

## MUSCLE GROUP EMPHASIZED

Chest ☐    Shoulders ☐    Back ☐    Arms ☐
Legs ☐    Abs ☐    None ☐

## WORKOUT QUALITY

Low ☐    Okay ☐    Good ☐    Great ☐

Post-Workout Mood and Energy: _____

_____

Post-Workout Food/Snack: _____

_____

_____

Notes: _____

_____

_____

_____

_____

_____

| MUSCLE GROUP | SET 1 | | SET 2 | | SET 3 | | SET 4 | | SET 5 | |
|---|---|---|---|---|---|---|---|---|---|---|
| EXERCISE | REPS | WGT | REPS | WGT | REPS | WGT | REPS | WGT | REPS | WGT |
| | | | | | | | | | | |
| | | | | | | | | | | |
| | | | | | | | | | | |
| | | | | | | | | | | |
| | | | | | | | | | | |
| | | | | | | | | | | |
| | | | | | | | | | | |
| | | | | | | | | | | |
| | | | | | | | | | | |
| | | | | | | | | | | |
| | | | | | | | | | | |
| | | | | | | | | | | |

Date: _____

Day of the Week: S ☐ M ☐ T ☐ W ☐ R ☐ F ☐ S ☐

Start Time: _____ Finish Time: _____

Stretch/Warm-Up: Yes ☐ No ☐

Cardio: _____ Level: _____

Pre-Workout Mood and Energy: _____

Pre-Workout Food/Snack: _____

## MUSCLE GROUP EMPHASIZED

Chest ☐ Shoulders ☐ Back ☐ Arms ☐
Legs ☐ Abs ☐ None ☐

## WORKOUT QUALITY

Low ☐ Okay ☐ Good ☐ Great ☐

Post-Workout Mood and Energy: _____

_____

Post-Workout Food/Snack: _____

_____

_____

Notes: _____

_____

_____

_____

_____

_____

| MUSCLE GROUP | SET 1 | | SET 2 | | SET 3 | | SET 4 | | SET 5 | |
|---|---|---|---|---|---|---|---|---|---|---|
| EXERCISE | REPS | WGT | REPS | WGT | REPS | WGT | REPS | WGT | REPS | WGT |
| | | | | | | | | | | |
| | | | | | | | | | | |
| | | | | | | | | | | |
| | | | | | | | | | | |
| | | | | | | | | | | |
| | | | | | | | | | | |
| | | | | | | | | | | |
| | | | | | | | | | | |
| | | | | | | | | | | |
| | | | | | | | | | | |
| | | | | | | | | | | |
| | | | | | | | | | | |

Date: _____

Day of the Week:  S ☐     M ☐     T ☐     W ☐     R ☐     F ☐     S ☐

Start Time: _____     Finish Time: _____

Stretch/Warm-Up:  Yes ☐     No ☐

Cardio: _____     Level: _____

Pre-Workout Mood and Energy: _____

Pre-Workout Food/Snack: _____

## MUSCLE GROUP EMPHASIZED

Chest ☐     Shoulders ☐     Back ☐     Arms ☐
Legs ☐     Abs ☐     None ☐

## WORKOUT QUALITY

Low ☐     Okay ☐     Good ☐     Great ☐

Post-Workout Mood and Energy: _____

_____

Post-Workout Food/Snack: _____

_____

_____

Notes: _____

_____

_____

_____

_____

_____

| MUSCLE GROUP | SET 1 | | SET 2 | | SET 3 | | SET 4 | | SET 5 | |
|---|---|---|---|---|---|---|---|---|---|---|
| EXERCISE | REPS | WGT | REPS | WGT | REPS | WGT | REPS | WGT | REPS | WGT |
| | | | | | | | | | | |
| | | | | | | | | | | |
| | | | | | | | | | | |
| | | | | | | | | | | |
| | | | | | | | | | | |
| | | | | | | | | | | |
| | | | | | | | | | | |
| | | | | | | | | | | |
| | | | | | | | | | | |
| | | | | | | | | | | |
| | | | | | | | | | | |

Date: _____

Day of the Week: S ☐   M ☐   T ☐   W ☐   R ☐   F ☐   S ☐

Start Time: _____   Finish Time: _____

Stretch/Warm-Up: Yes ☐   No ☐

Cardio: _____   Level: _____

Pre-Workout Mood and Energy: _____

Pre-Workout Food/Snack: _____

## MUSCLE GROUP EMPHASIZED

Chest ☐   Shoulders ☐   Back ☐   Arms ☐
Legs ☐   Abs ☐   None ☐

## WORKOUT QUALITY

Low ☐   Okay ☐   Good ☐   Great ☐

Post-Workout Mood and Energy: _____

_____

Post-Workout Food/Snack: _____

_____

_____

Notes: _____

_____

_____

_____

_____

_____

| MUSCLE GROUP | SET 1 | | SET 2 | | SET 3 | | SET 4 | | SET 5 | |
|---|---|---|---|---|---|---|---|---|---|---|
| EXERCISE | REPS | WGT | REPS | WGT | REPS | WGT | REPS | WGT | REPS | WGT |
| | | | | | | | | | | |
| | | | | | | | | | | |
| | | | | | | | | | | |
| | | | | | | | | | | |
| | | | | | | | | | | |
| | | | | | | | | | | |
| | | | | | | | | | | |
| | | | | | | | | | | |
| | | | | | | | | | | |
| | | | | | | | | | | |
| | | | | | | | | | | |
| | | | | | | | | | | |

Date: _____

Day of the Week: S ☐    M ☐    T ☐    W ☐    R ☐    F ☐    S ☐

Start Time: _____    Finish Time: _____

Stretch/Warm-Up: Yes ☐    No ☐

Cardio: _____    Level: _____

Pre-Workout Mood and Energy: _____

Pre-Workout Food/Snack: _____

## MUSCLE GROUP EMPHASIZED

Chest ☐    Shoulders ☐    Back ☐    Arms ☐
Legs ☐    Abs ☐    None ☐

## WORKOUT QUALITY

Low ☐    Okay ☐    Good ☐    Great ☐

Post-Workout Mood and Energy: _____

_____

Post-Workout Food/Snack: _____

_____

_____

Notes: _____

_____

_____

_____

_____

_____

| MUSCLE GROUP | SET 1 | | SET 2 | | SET 3 | | SET 4 | | SET 5 | |
|---|---|---|---|---|---|---|---|---|---|---|
| EXERCISE | REPS | WGT | REPS | WGT | REPS | WGT | REPS | WGT | REPS | WGT |
| | | | | | | | | | | |
| | | | | | | | | | | |
| | | | | | | | | | | |
| | | | | | | | | | | |
| | | | | | | | | | | |
| | | | | | | | | | | |
| | | | | | | | | | | |
| | | | | | | | | | | |
| | | | | | | | | | | |
| | | | | | | | | | | |
| | | | | | | | | | | |
| | | | | | | | | | | |

Date: _____

Day of the Week:  S ☐     M ☐     T ☐     W ☐     R ☐     F ☐     S ☐

Start Time: _____     Finish Time: _____

Stretch/Warm-Up:  Yes ☐     No ☐

Cardio: _____     Level: _____

Pre-Workout Mood and Energy: _____

Pre-Workout Food/Snack: _____

## MUSCLE GROUP EMPHASIZED

Chest ☐     Shoulders ☐     Back ☐     Arms ☐
Legs ☐     Abs ☐     None ☐

## WORKOUT QUALITY

Low ☐     Okay ☐     Good ☐     Great ☐

Post-Workout Mood and Energy: _____

_____

Post-Workout Food/Snack: _____

_____

_____

Notes: _____

_____

_____

_____

_____

_____

| MUSCLE GROUP | SET 1 | | SET 2 | | SET 3 | | SET 4 | | SET 5 | |
|---|---|---|---|---|---|---|---|---|---|---|
| **EXERCISE** | REPS | WGT | REPS | WGT | REPS | WGT | REPS | WGT | REPS | WGT |
| | | | | | | | | | | |
| | | | | | | | | | | |
| | | | | | | | | | | |
| | | | | | | | | | | |
| | | | | | | | | | | |
| | | | | | | | | | | |
| | | | | | | | | | | |
| | | | | | | | | | | |
| | | | | | | | | | | |
| | | | | | | | | | | |
| | | | | | | | | | | |
| | | | | | | | | | | |

Date: _____

Day of the Week:  S ☐   M ☐   T ☐   W ☐   R ☐   F ☐   S ☐

Start Time: _____   Finish Time: _____

Stretch/Warm-Up:  Yes ☐   No ☐

Cardio: _____   Level: _____

Pre-Workout Mood and Energy: _____

Pre-Workout Food/Snack: _____

## MUSCLE GROUP EMPHASIZED

Chest ☐   Shoulders ☐   Back ☐   Arms ☐
Legs ☐   Abs ☐   None ☐

## WORKOUT QUALITY

Low ☐   Okay ☐   Good ☐   Great ☐

Post-Workout Mood and Energy: _____

_____

Post-Workout Food/Snack: _____

_____

_____

Notes: _____

_____

_____

_____

_____

_____

| MUSCLE GROUP | SET 1 | | SET 2 | | SET 3 | | SET 4 | | SET 5 | |
|---|---|---|---|---|---|---|---|---|---|---|
| EXERCISE | REPS | WGT | REPS | WGT | REPS | WGT | REPS | WGT | REPS | WGT |
| | | | | | | | | | | |
| | | | | | | | | | | |
| | | | | | | | | | | |
| | | | | | | | | | | |
| | | | | | | | | | | |
| | | | | | | | | | | |
| | | | | | | | | | | |
| | | | | | | | | | | |
| | | | | | | | | | | |
| | | | | | | | | | | |
| | | | | | | | | | | |

Date: _____

Day of the Week: S ☐  M ☐  T ☐  W ☐  R ☐  F ☐  S ☐

Start Time: _____  Finish Time: _____

Stretch/Warm-Up: Yes ☐  No ☐

Cardio: _____  Level: _____

Pre-Workout Mood and Energy: _____

Pre-Workout Food/Snack: _____

## MUSCLE GROUP EMPHASIZED

Chest ☐  Shoulders ☐  Back ☐  Arms ☐
Legs ☐  Abs ☐  None ☐

## WORKOUT QUALITY

Low ☐  Okay ☐  Good ☐  Great ☐

Post-Workout Mood and Energy: _____

_____

Post-Workout Food/Snack: _____

_____

_____

Notes: _____

_____

_____

_____

_____

_____

| MUSCLE GROUP | SET 1 | | SET 2 | | SET 3 | | SET 4 | | SET 5 | |
|---|---|---|---|---|---|---|---|---|---|---|
| EXERCISE | REPS | WGT | REPS | WGT | REPS | WGT | REPS | WGT | REPS | WGT |
| | | | | | | | | | | |
| | | | | | | | | | | |
| | | | | | | | | | | |
| | | | | | | | | | | |
| | | | | | | | | | | |
| | | | | | | | | | | |
| | | | | | | | | | | |
| | | | | | | | | | | |
| | | | | | | | | | | |
| | | | | | | | | | | |
| | | | | | | | | | | |
| | | | | | | | | | | |
| | | | | | | | | | | |

Date: _____

Day of the Week:  S ☐    M ☐    T ☐    W ☐    R ☐    F ☐    S ☐

Start Time: _____    Finish Time: _____

Stretch/Warm-Up:  Yes ☐    No ☐

Cardio: _____    Level: _____

Pre-Workout Mood and Energy: _____

Pre-Workout Food/Snack: _____

## MUSCLE GROUP EMPHASIZED

Chest ☐    Shoulders ☐    Back ☐    Arms ☐
Legs ☐    Abs ☐    None ☐

## WORKOUT QUALITY

Low ☐    Okay ☐    Good ☐    Great ☐

Post-Workout Mood and Energy: _____

_____

Post-Workout Food/Snack: _____

_____

_____

Notes: _____

_____

_____

_____

_____

_____

| MUSCLE GROUP | SET 1 | | SET 2 | | SET 3 | | SET 4 | | SET 5 | |
|---|---|---|---|---|---|---|---|---|---|---|
| EXERCISE | REPS | WGT | REPS | WGT | REPS | WGT | REPS | WGT | REPS | WGT |
| | | | | | | | | | | |
| | | | | | | | | | | |
| | | | | | | | | | | |
| | | | | | | | | | | |
| | | | | | | | | | | |
| | | | | | | | | | | |
| | | | | | | | | | | |
| | | | | | | | | | | |
| | | | | | | | | | | |
| | | | | | | | | | | |
| | | | | | | | | | | |

Date: _____

Day of the Week:  S ☐   M ☐   T ☐   W ☐   R ☐   F ☐   S ☐

Start Time: _____   Finish Time: _____

Stretch/Warm-Up:  Yes ☐    No ☐

Cardio: _____   Level: _____

Pre-Workout Mood and Energy: _____

Pre-Workout Food/Snack: _____

## MUSCLE GROUP EMPHASIZED

Chest ☐    Shoulders ☐    Back ☐    Arms ☐
Legs ☐    Abs ☐    None ☐

## WORKOUT QUALITY

Low ☐    Okay ☐    Good ☐    Great ☐

Post-Workout Mood and Energy: _____

_____

Post-Workout Food/Snack: _____

_____

_____

Notes: _____

_____

_____

_____

_____

_____

| MUSCLE GROUP | SET 1 | | SET 2 | | SET 3 | | SET 4 | | SET 5 | |
|---|---|---|---|---|---|---|---|---|---|---|
| EXERCISE | REPS | WGT | REPS | WGT | REPS | WGT | REPS | WGT | REPS | WGT |
| | | | | | | | | | | |
| | | | | | | | | | | |
| | | | | | | | | | | |
| | | | | | | | | | | |
| | | | | | | | | | | |
| | | | | | | | | | | |
| | | | | | | | | | | |
| | | | | | | | | | | |
| | | | | | | | | | | |
| | | | | | | | | | | |
| | | | | | | | | | | |
| | | | | | | | | | | |

Date: _____

Day of the Week:  S ☐    M ☐    T ☐    W ☐    R ☐    F ☐    S ☐

Start Time: _____    Finish Time: _____

Stretch/Warm-Up:  Yes ☐    No ☐

Cardio: _____    Level: _____

Pre-Workout Mood and Energy: _____

Pre-Workout Food/Snack: _____

## MUSCLE GROUP EMPHASIZED

Chest ☐    Shoulders ☐    Back ☐    Arms ☐
Legs ☐    Abs ☐    None ☐

## WORKOUT QUALITY

Low ☐    Okay ☐    Good ☐    Great ☐

Post-Workout Mood and Energy: _____

_____

Post-Workout Food/Snack: _____

_____

_____

Notes: _____

_____

_____

_____

_____

_____

| MUSCLE GROUP | SET 1 | | SET 2 | | SET 3 | | SET 4 | | SET 5 | |
|---|---|---|---|---|---|---|---|---|---|---|
| EXERCISE | REPS | WGT | REPS | WGT | REPS | WGT | REPS | WGT | REPS | WGT |
| | | | | | | | | | | |
| | | | | | | | | | | |
| | | | | | | | | | | |
| | | | | | | | | | | |
| | | | | | | | | | | |
| | | | | | | | | | | |
| | | | | | | | | | | |
| | | | | | | | | | | |
| | | | | | | | | | | |
| | | | | | | | | | | |
| | | | | | | | | | | |

Date: _____

Day of the Week:  S ☐    M ☐    T ☐    W ☐    R ☐    F ☐    S ☐

Start Time: _____    Finish Time: _____

Stretch/Warm-Up:  Yes ☐    No ☐

Cardio: _____    Level: _____

Pre-Workout Mood and Energy: _____

Pre-Workout Food/Snack: _____

## MUSCLE GROUP EMPHASIZED

Chest ☐    Shoulders ☐    Back ☐    Arms ☐
Legs ☐    Abs ☐    None ☐

## WORKOUT QUALITY

Low ☐    Okay ☐    Good ☐    Great ☐

Post-Workout Mood and Energy: _____

_____

Post-Workout Food/Snack: _____

_____

_____

Notes: _____

_____

_____

_____

_____

_____

| MUSCLE GROUP | SET 1 | | SET 2 | | SET 3 | | SET 4 | | SET 5 | |
| --- | --- | --- | --- | --- | --- | --- | --- | --- | --- | --- |
| EXERCISE | REPS | WGT | REPS | WGT | REPS | WGT | REPS | WGT | REPS | WGT |
| | | | | | | | | | | |
| | | | | | | | | | | |
| | | | | | | | | | | |
| | | | | | | | | | | |
| | | | | | | | | | | |
| | | | | | | | | | | |
| | | | | | | | | | | |
| | | | | | | | | | | |
| | | | | | | | | | | |
| | | | | | | | | | | |
| | | | | | | | | | | |
| | | | | | | | | | | |

Date: _____

Day of the Week:  S ☐    M ☐    T ☐    W ☐    R ☐    F ☐    S ☐

Start Time: _____    Finish Time: _____

Stretch/Warm-Up:  Yes ☐    No ☐

Cardio: _____    Level: _____

Pre-Workout Mood and Energy: _____

Pre-Workout Food/Snack: _____

## MUSCLE GROUP EMPHASIZED

Chest ☐    Shoulders ☐    Back ☐    Arms ☐
Legs ☐    Abs ☐    None ☐

## WORKOUT QUALITY

Low ☐    Okay ☐    Good ☐    Great ☐

Post-Workout Mood and Energy: _____

_____

Post-Workout Food/Snack: _____

_____

_____

Notes: _____

_____

_____

_____

_____

_____

| MUSCLE GROUP | SET 1 | | SET 2 | | SET 3 | | SET 4 | | SET 5 | |
|---|---|---|---|---|---|---|---|---|---|---|
| **EXERCISE** | **REPS** | **WGT** | **REPS** | **WGT** | **REPS** | **WGT** | **REPS** | **WGT** | **REPS** | **WGT** |
| | | | | | | | | | | |
| | | | | | | | | | | |
| | | | | | | | | | | |
| | | | | | | | | | | |
| | | | | | | | | | | |
| | | | | | | | | | | |
| | | | | | | | | | | |
| | | | | | | | | | | |
| | | | | | | | | | | |
| | | | | | | | | | | |
| | | | | | | | | | | |
| | | | | | | | | | | |

Date: _____

Day of the Week:  S ☐   M ☐   T ☐   W ☐   R ☐   F ☐   S ☐

Start Time: _____   Finish Time: _____

Stretch/Warm-Up:  Yes ☐   No ☐

Cardio: _____   Level: _____

Pre-Workout Mood and Energy: _____

Pre-Workout Food/Snack: _____

### MUSCLE GROUP EMPHASIZED

Chest ☐   Shoulders ☐   Back ☐   Arms ☐
Legs ☐   Abs ☐   None ☐

### WORKOUT QUALITY

Low ☐   Okay ☐   Good ☐   Great ☐

Post-Workout Mood and Energy: _____

_____

Post-Workout Food/Snack: _____

_____

_____

Notes: _____

_____

_____

_____

_____

_____

| MUSCLE GROUP | SET 1 | | SET 2 | | SET 3 | | SET 4 | | SET 5 | |
|---|---|---|---|---|---|---|---|---|---|---|
| EXERCISE | REPS | WGT | REPS | WGT | REPS | WGT | REPS | WGT | REPS | WGT |
| | | | | | | | | | | |
| | | | | | | | | | | |
| | | | | | | | | | | |
| | | | | | | | | | | |
| | | | | | | | | | | |
| | | | | | | | | | | |
| | | | | | | | | | | |
| | | | | | | | | | | |
| | | | | | | | | | | |
| | | | | | | | | | | |
| | | | | | | | | | | |

Date: _____

Day of the Week:  S ☐   M ☐   T ☐   W ☐   R ☐   F ☐   S ☐

Start Time: _____    Finish Time: _____

Stretch/Warm-Up:  Yes ☐    No ☐

Cardio: _____    Level: _____

Pre-Workout Mood and Energy: _____

Pre-Workout Food/Snack: _____

## MUSCLE GROUP EMPHASIZED

Chest ☐    Shoulders ☐    Back ☐    Arms ☐
Legs ☐    Abs ☐    None ☐

## WORKOUT QUALITY

Low ☐    Okay ☐    Good ☐    Great ☐

Post-Workout Mood and Energy: _____

_____

Post-Workout Food/Snack: _____

_____

_____

Notes: _____

_____

_____

_____

_____

| MUSCLE GROUP | SET 1 | | SET 2 | | SET 3 | | SET 4 | | SET 5 | |
|---|---|---|---|---|---|---|---|---|---|---|
| **EXERCISE** | REPS | WGT | REPS | WGT | REPS | WGT | REPS | WGT | REPS | WGT |
| | | | | | | | | | | |
| | | | | | | | | | | |
| | | | | | | | | | | |
| | | | | | | | | | | |
| | | | | | | | | | | |
| | | | | | | | | | | |
| | | | | | | | | | | |
| | | | | | | | | | | |
| | | | | | | | | | | |
| | | | | | | | | | | |
| | | | | | | | | | | |
| | | | | | | | | | | |

Date: _____

Day of the Week: S ☐   M ☐   T ☐   W ☐   R ☐   F ☐   S ☐

Start Time: _____   Finish Time: _____

Stretch/Warm-Up: Yes ☐   No ☐

Cardio: _____   Level: _____

Pre-Workout Mood and Energy: _____

Pre-Workout Food/Snack: _____

## MUSCLE GROUP EMPHASIZED

Chest ☐   Shoulders ☐   Back ☐   Arms ☐
Legs ☐   Abs ☐   None ☐

## WORKOUT QUALITY

Low ☐   Okay ☐   Good ☐   Great ☐

Post-Workout Mood and Energy: _____

_____

Post-Workout Food/Snack: _____

_____

_____

Notes: _____

_____

_____

_____

_____

_____

| MUSCLE GROUP | SET 1 | | SET 2 | | SET 3 | | SET 4 | | SET 5 | |
|---|---|---|---|---|---|---|---|---|---|---|
| EXERCISE | REPS | WGT | REPS | WGT | REPS | WGT | REPS | WGT | REPS | WGT |
| | | | | | | | | | | |
| | | | | | | | | | | |
| | | | | | | | | | | |
| | | | | | | | | | | |
| | | | | | | | | | | |
| | | | | | | | | | | |
| | | | | | | | | | | |
| | | | | | | | | | | |
| | | | | | | | | | | |
| | | | | | | | | | | |
| | | | | | | | | | | |
| | | | | | | | | | | |

Date: _____

Day of the Week:  S ☐    M ☐    T ☐    W ☐    R ☐    F ☐    S ☐

Start Time: _____    Finish Time: _____

Stretch/Warm-Up:  Yes ☐    No ☐

Cardio: _____    Level: _____

Pre-Workout Mood and Energy: _____

Pre-Workout Food/Snack: _____

## MUSCLE GROUP EMPHASIZED

Chest ☐    Shoulders ☐    Back ☐    Arms ☐
Legs ☐    Abs ☐    None ☐

## WORKOUT QUALITY

Low ☐    Okay ☐    Good ☐    Great ☐

Post-Workout Mood and Energy: _____

_____

Post-Workout Food/Snack: _____

_____

_____

Notes: _____

_____

_____

_____

_____

_____

| MUSCLE GROUP | SET 1 | | SET 2 | | SET 3 | | SET 4 | | SET 5 | |
|---|---|---|---|---|---|---|---|---|---|---|
| EXERCISE | REPS | WGT | REPS | WGT | REPS | WGT | REPS | WGT | REPS | WGT |
| | | | | | | | | | | |
| | | | | | | | | | | |
| | | | | | | | | | | |
| | | | | | | | | | | |
| | | | | | | | | | | |
| | | | | | | | | | | |
| | | | | | | | | | | |
| | | | | | | | | | | |
| | | | | | | | | | | |
| | | | | | | | | | | |
| | | | | | | | | | | |
| | | | | | | | | | | |

Date: _____

Day of the Week:  S ☐   M ☐   T ☐   W ☐   R ☐   F ☐   S ☐

Start Time: _____     Finish Time: _____

Stretch/Warm-Up:  Yes ☐    No ☐

Cardio: _____     Level: _____

Pre-Workout Mood and Energy: _____

Pre-Workout Food/Snack: _____

## MUSCLE GROUP EMPHASIZED

Chest ☐   Shoulders ☐   Back ☐   Arms ☐
Legs ☐   Abs ☐   None ☐

## WORKOUT QUALITY

Low ☐   Okay ☐   Good ☐   Great ☐

Post-Workout Mood and Energy: _____

_____

Post-Workout Food/Snack: _____

_____

_____

Notes: _____

_____

_____

_____

_____

_____

| MUSCLE GROUP | SET 1 | | SET 2 | | SET 3 | | SET 4 | | SET 5 | |
|---|---|---|---|---|---|---|---|---|---|---|
| EXERCISE | REPS | WGT | REPS | WGT | REPS | WGT | REPS | WGT | REPS | WGT |
| | | | | | | | | | | |
| | | | | | | | | | | |
| | | | | | | | | | | |
| | | | | | | | | | | |
| | | | | | | | | | | |
| | | | | | | | | | | |
| | | | | | | | | | | |
| | | | | | | | | | | |
| | | | | | | | | | | |
| | | | | | | | | | | |
| | | | | | | | | | | |
| | | | | | | | | | | |

Date: _____

Day of the Week:  S ☐    M ☐    T ☐    W ☐    R ☐    F ☐    S ☐

Start Time: _____    Finish Time: _____

Stretch/Warm-Up:  Yes ☐    No ☐

Cardio: _____    Level: _____

Pre-Workout Mood and Energy: _____

Pre-Workout Food/Snack: _____

## MUSCLE GROUP EMPHASIZED

Chest ☐    Shoulders ☐    Back ☐    Arms ☐
Legs ☐    Abs ☐    None ☐

## WORKOUT QUALITY

Low ☐    Okay ☐    Good ☐    Great ☐

Post-Workout Mood and Energy: _____

_____

Post-Workout Food/Snack: _____

_____

_____

Notes: _____

_____

_____

_____

_____

_____

| MUSCLE GROUP | SET 1 | | SET 2 | | SET 3 | | SET 4 | | SET 5 | |
|---|---|---|---|---|---|---|---|---|---|---|
| EXERCISE | REPS | WGT | REPS | WGT | REPS | WGT | REPS | WGT | REPS | WGT |
| | | | | | | | | | | |
| | | | | | | | | | | |
| | | | | | | | | | | |
| | | | | | | | | | | |
| | | | | | | | | | | |
| | | | | | | | | | | |
| | | | | | | | | | | |
| | | | | | | | | | | |
| | | | | | | | | | | |
| | | | | | | | | | | |
| | | | | | | | | | | |
| | | | | | | | | | | |

Date: _____

Day of the Week:  S ☐    M ☐    T ☐    W ☐    R ☐    F ☐    S ☐

Start Time: _____    Finish Time: _____

Stretch/Warm-Up:  Yes ☐    No ☐

Cardio: _____    Level: _____

Pre-Workout Mood and Energy: _____

Pre-Workout Food/Snack: _____

## MUSCLE GROUP EMPHASIZED

Chest ☐    Shoulders ☐    Back ☐    Arms ☐
Legs ☐    Abs ☐    None ☐

## WORKOUT QUALITY

Low ☐    Okay ☐    Good ☐    Great ☐

Post-Workout Mood and Energy: _____

_____

Post-Workout Food/Snack: _____

_____

_____

Notes: _____

_____

_____

_____

_____

_____

| MUSCLE GROUP | SET 1 | | SET 2 | | SET 3 | | SET 4 | | SET 5 | |
|---|---|---|---|---|---|---|---|---|---|---|
| EXERCISE | REPS | WGT | REPS | WGT | REPS | WGT | REPS | WGT | REPS | WGT |
| | | | | | | | | | | |
| | | | | | | | | | | |
| | | | | | | | | | | |
| | | | | | | | | | | |
| | | | | | | | | | | |
| | | | | | | | | | | |
| | | | | | | | | | | |
| | | | | | | | | | | |
| | | | | | | | | | | |
| | | | | | | | | | | |
| | | | | | | | | | | |
| | | | | | | | | | | |
| | | | | | | | | | | |

Date: _____

Day of the Week:  S ☐   M ☐   T ☐   W ☐   R ☐   F ☐   S ☐

Start Time: _____   Finish Time: _____

Stretch/Warm-Up:  Yes ☐   No ☐

Cardio: _____   Level: _____

Pre-Workout Mood and Energy: _____

Pre-Workout Food/Snack: _____

## MUSCLE GROUP EMPHASIZED

Chest ☐   Shoulders ☐   Back ☐   Arms ☐
Legs ☐   Abs ☐   None ☐

## WORKOUT QUALITY

Low ☐   Okay ☐   Good ☐   Great ☐

Post-Workout Mood and Energy: _____

_____

Post-Workout Food/Snack: _____

_____

_____

Notes: _____

_____

_____

_____

_____

_____

| MUSCLE GROUP | SET 1 | | SET 2 | | SET 3 | | SET 4 | | SET 5 | |
| --- | --- | --- | --- | --- | --- | --- | --- | --- | --- | --- |
| EXERCISE | REPS | WGT | REPS | WGT | REPS | WGT | REPS | WGT | REPS | WGT |
| | | | | | | | | | | |
| | | | | | | | | | | |
| | | | | | | | | | | |
| | | | | | | | | | | |
| | | | | | | | | | | |
| | | | | | | | | | | |
| | | | | | | | | | | |
| | | | | | | | | | | |
| | | | | | | | | | | |
| | | | | | | | | | | |
| | | | | | | | | | | |

Date: _____

Day of the Week: S ☐   M ☐   T ☐   W ☐   R ☐   F ☐   S ☐

Start Time: _____   Finish Time: _____

Stretch/Warm-Up: Yes ☐   No ☐

Cardio: _____   Level: _____

Pre-Workout Mood and Energy: _____

Pre-Workout Food/Snack: _____

## MUSCLE GROUP EMPHASIZED

Chest ☐   Shoulders ☐   Back ☐   Arms ☐
Legs ☐   Abs ☐   None ☐

## WORKOUT QUALITY

Low ☐   Okay ☐   Good ☐   Great ☐

Post-Workout Mood and Energy: _____

_____

Post-Workout Food/Snack: _____

_____

_____

Notes: _____

_____

_____

_____

_____

_____

| MUSCLE GROUP | SET 1 | | SET 2 | | SET 3 | | SET 4 | | SET 5 | |
|---|---|---|---|---|---|---|---|---|---|---|
| EXERCISE | REPS | WGT | REPS | WGT | REPS | WGT | REPS | WGT | REPS | WGT |
| | | | | | | | | | | |
| | | | | | | | | | | |
| | | | | | | | | | | |
| | | | | | | | | | | |
| | | | | | | | | | | |
| | | | | | | | | | | |
| | | | | | | | | | | |
| | | | | | | | | | | |
| | | | | | | | | | | |
| | | | | | | | | | | |
| | | | | | | | | | | |

Date: _____

Day of the Week: S ☐   M ☐   T ☐   W ☐   R ☐   F ☐   S ☐

Start Time: _____   Finish Time: _____

Stretch/Warm-Up: Yes ☐   No ☐

Cardio: _____   Level: _____

Pre-Workout Mood and Energy: _____

Pre-Workout Food/Snack: _____

### MUSCLE GROUP EMPHASIZED

Chest ☐   Shoulders ☐   Back ☐   Arms ☐
Legs ☐   Abs ☐   None ☐

### WORKOUT QUALITY

Low ☐   Okay ☐   Good ☐   Great ☐

Post-Workout Mood and Energy: _____

_____

Post-Workout Food/Snack: _____

_____

_____

Notes: _____

_____

_____

_____

_____

_____

| MUSCLE GROUP | SET 1 | | SET 2 | | SET 3 | | SET 4 | | SET 5 | |
|---|---|---|---|---|---|---|---|---|---|---|
| EXERCISE | REPS | WGT | REPS | WGT | REPS | WGT | REPS | WGT | REPS | WGT |
| | | | | | | | | | | |
| | | | | | | | | | | |
| | | | | | | | | | | |
| | | | | | | | | | | |
| | | | | | | | | | | |
| | | | | | | | | | | |
| | | | | | | | | | | |
| | | | | | | | | | | |
| | | | | | | | | | | |
| | | | | | | | | | | |
| | | | | | | | | | | |

Date: _____

Day of the Week:  S ☐    M ☐    T ☐    W ☐    R ☐    F ☐    S ☐

Start Time: _____    Finish Time: _____

Stretch/Warm-Up:  Yes ☐    No ☐

Cardio: _____    Level: _____

Pre-Workout Mood and Energy: _____

Pre-Workout Food/Snack: _____

## MUSCLE GROUP EMPHASIZED

Chest ☐    Shoulders ☐    Back ☐    Arms ☐
Legs ☐    Abs ☐    None ☐

## WORKOUT QUALITY

Low ☐    Okay ☐    Good ☐    Great ☐

Post-Workout Mood and Energy: _____

_____

Post-Workout Food/Snack: _____

_____

_____

Notes: _____

_____

_____

_____

_____

_____

| MUSCLE GROUP | SET 1 | | SET 2 | | SET 3 | | SET 4 | | SET 5 | |
| --- | --- | --- | --- | --- | --- | --- | --- | --- | --- | --- |
| EXERCISE | REPS | WGT | REPS | WGT | REPS | WGT | REPS | WGT | REPS | WGT |
| | | | | | | | | | | |
| | | | | | | | | | | |
| | | | | | | | | | | |
| | | | | | | | | | | |
| | | | | | | | | | | |
| | | | | | | | | | | |
| | | | | | | | | | | |
| | | | | | | | | | | |
| | | | | | | | | | | |
| | | | | | | | | | | |
| | | | | | | | | | | |

Date: _____

Day of the Week:  S ☐   M ☐   T ☐   W ☐   R ☐   F ☐   S ☐

Start Time: _____   Finish Time: _____

Stretch/Warm-Up:  Yes ☐   No ☐

Cardio: _____   Level: _____

Pre-Workout Mood and Energy: _____

Pre-Workout Food/Snack: _____

## MUSCLE GROUP EMPHASIZED

Chest ☐   Shoulders ☐   Back ☐   Arms ☐
Legs ☐   Abs ☐   None ☐

## WORKOUT QUALITY

Low ☐   Okay ☐   Good ☐   Great ☐

Post-Workout Mood and Energy: _____

_____

Post-Workout Food/Snack: _____

_____

_____

Notes: _____

_____

_____

_____

_____

_____

| MUSCLE GROUP | SET 1 | | SET 2 | | SET 3 | | SET 4 | | SET 5 | |
|---|---|---|---|---|---|---|---|---|---|---|
| EXERCISE | REPS | WGT | REPS | WGT | REPS | WGT | REPS | WGT | REPS | WGT |
| | | | | | | | | | | |
| | | | | | | | | | | |
| | | | | | | | | | | |
| | | | | | | | | | | |
| | | | | | | | | | | |
| | | | | | | | | | | |
| | | | | | | | | | | |
| | | | | | | | | | | |
| | | | | | | | | | | |
| | | | | | | | | | | |
| | | | | | | | | | | |
| | | | | | | | | | | |

Date: _____

Day of the Week:  S ☐    M ☐    T ☐    W ☐    R ☐    F ☐    S ☐

Start Time: _____    Finish Time: _____

Stretch/Warm-Up:  Yes ☐    No ☐

Cardio: _____    Level: _____

Pre-Workout Mood and Energy: _____

Pre-Workout Food/Snack: _____

## MUSCLE GROUP EMPHASIZED

Chest ☐    Shoulders ☐    Back ☐    Arms ☐
Legs ☐    Abs ☐    None ☐

## WORKOUT QUALITY

Low ☐    Okay ☐    Good ☐    Great ☐

Post-Workout Mood and Energy: _____

_____

Post-Workout Food/Snack: _____

_____

_____

Notes: _____

_____

_____

_____

_____

_____

| MUSCLE GROUP | SET 1 | | SET 2 | | SET 3 | | SET 4 | | SET 5 | |
|---|---|---|---|---|---|---|---|---|---|---|
| EXERCISE | REPS | WGT | REPS | WGT | REPS | WGT | REPS | WGT | REPS | WGT |
| | | | | | | | | | | |
| | | | | | | | | | | |
| | | | | | | | | | | |
| | | | | | | | | | | |
| | | | | | | | | | | |
| | | | | | | | | | | |
| | | | | | | | | | | |
| | | | | | | | | | | |
| | | | | | | | | | | |
| | | | | | | | | | | |
| | | | | | | | | | | |
| | | | | | | | | | | |

Date: _____

Day of the Week:  S ☐    M ☐    T ☐    W ☐    R ☐    F ☐    S ☐

Start Time: _____    Finish Time: _____

Stretch/Warm-Up: Yes ☐    No ☐

Cardio: _____    Level: _____

Pre-Workout Mood and Energy: _____

Pre-Workout Food/Snack: _____

## MUSCLE GROUP EMPHASIZED

Chest ☐    Shoulders ☐    Back ☐    Arms ☐
Legs ☐    Abs ☐    None ☐

## WORKOUT QUALITY

Low ☐    Okay ☐    Good ☐    Great ☐

Post-Workout Mood and Energy: _____

_____

Post-Workout Food/Snack: _____

_____

_____

Notes: _____

_____

_____

_____

_____

_____

| MUSCLE GROUP | SET 1 | | SET 2 | | SET 3 | | SET 4 | | SET 5 | |
|---|---|---|---|---|---|---|---|---|---|---|
| EXERCISE | REPS | WGT | REPS | WGT | REPS | WGT | REPS | WGT | REPS | WGT |
| | | | | | | | | | | |
| | | | | | | | | | | |
| | | | | | | | | | | |
| | | | | | | | | | | |
| | | | | | | | | | | |
| | | | | | | | | | | |
| | | | | | | | | | | |
| | | | | | | | | | | |
| | | | | | | | | | | |
| | | | | | | | | | | |
| | | | | | | | | | | |
| | | | | | | | | | | |

Date: _____

Day of the Week: S ☐   M ☐   T ☐   W ☐   R ☐   F ☐   S ☐

Start Time: _____   Finish Time: _____

Stretch/Warm-Up: Yes ☐   No ☐

Cardio: _____   Level: _____

Pre-Workout Mood and Energy: _____

Pre-Workout Food/Snack: _____

### MUSCLE GROUP EMPHASIZED

Chest ☐   Shoulders ☐   Back ☐   Arms ☐
Legs ☐   Abs ☐   None ☐

### WORKOUT QUALITY

Low ☐   Okay ☐   Good ☐   Great ☐

Post-Workout Mood and Energy: _____

_____

Post-Workout Food/Snack: _____

_____

_____

Notes: _____

_____

_____

_____

_____

_____

| MUSCLE GROUP | SET 1 | | SET 2 | | SET 3 | | SET 4 | | SET 5 | |
|---|---|---|---|---|---|---|---|---|---|---|
| EXERCISE | REPS | WGT | REPS | WGT | REPS | WGT | REPS | WGT | REPS | WGT |
| | | | | | | | | | | |
| | | | | | | | | | | |
| | | | | | | | | | | |
| | | | | | | | | | | |
| | | | | | | | | | | |
| | | | | | | | | | | |
| | | | | | | | | | | |
| | | | | | | | | | | |
| | | | | | | | | | | |
| | | | | | | | | | | |
| | | | | | | | | | | |

Date: _____

Day of the Week:  S ☐     M ☐     T ☐     W ☐     R ☐     F ☐     S ☐

Start Time: _____     Finish Time: _____

Stretch/Warm-Up:  Yes ☐     No ☐

Cardio: _____     Level: _____

Pre-Workout Mood and Energy: _____

Pre-Workout Food/Snack: _____

## MUSCLE GROUP EMPHASIZED

Chest ☐     Shoulders ☐     Back ☐     Arms ☐
Legs ☐     Abs ☐     None ☐

## WORKOUT QUALITY

Low ☐     Okay ☐     Good ☐     Great ☐

Post-Workout Mood and Energy: _____

_____

Post-Workout Food/Snack: _____

_____

_____

Notes: _____

_____

_____

_____

_____

_____

| MUSCLE GROUP | SET 1 | | SET 2 | | SET 3 | | SET 4 | | SET 5 | |
|---|---|---|---|---|---|---|---|---|---|---|
| EXERCISE | REPS | WGT | REPS | WGT | REPS | WGT | REPS | WGT | REPS | WGT |
| | | | | | | | | | | |
| | | | | | | | | | | |
| | | | | | | | | | | |
| | | | | | | | | | | |
| | | | | | | | | | | |
| | | | | | | | | | | |
| | | | | | | | | | | |
| | | | | | | | | | | |
| | | | | | | | | | | |
| | | | | | | | | | | |
| | | | | | | | | | | |

Date: _____

Day of the Week:  S ☐    M ☐    T ☐    W ☐    R ☐    F ☐    S ☐

Start Time: _____    Finish Time: _____

Stretch/Warm-Up:  Yes ☐    No ☐

Cardio: _____    Level: _____

Pre-Workout Mood and Energy: _____

Pre-Workout Food/Snack: _____

## MUSCLE GROUP EMPHASIZED
Chest ☐    Shoulders ☐    Back ☐    Arms ☐
Legs ☐    Abs ☐    None ☐

## WORKOUT QUALITY
Low ☐    Okay ☐    Good ☐    Great ☐

Post-Workout Mood and Energy: _____

_____

Post-Workout Food/Snack: _____

_____

_____

Notes: _____

_____

_____

_____

_____

_____

| MUSCLE GROUP | SET 1 | | SET 2 | | SET 3 | | SET 4 | | SET 5 | |
|---|---|---|---|---|---|---|---|---|---|---|
| EXERCISE | REPS | WGT | REPS | WGT | REPS | WGT | REPS | WGT | REPS | WGT |
| | | | | | | | | | | |
| | | | | | | | | | | |
| | | | | | | | | | | |
| | | | | | | | | | | |
| | | | | | | | | | | |
| | | | | | | | | | | |
| | | | | | | | | | | |
| | | | | | | | | | | |
| | | | | | | | | | | |
| | | | | | | | | | | |
| | | | | | | | | | | |
| | | | | | | | | | | |

Date: _____

Day of the Week:  S ☐    M ☐    T ☐    W ☐    R ☐    F ☐    S ☐

Start Time: _____    Finish Time: _____

Stretch/Warm-Up:  Yes ☐    No ☐

Cardio: _____    Level: _____

Pre-Workout Mood and Energy: _____

Pre-Workout Food/Snack: _____

## MUSCLE GROUP EMPHASIZED

Chest ☐    Shoulders ☐    Back ☐    Arms ☐
Legs ☐    Abs ☐    None ☐

## WORKOUT QUALITY

Low ☐    Okay ☐    Good ☐    Great ☐

Post-Workout Mood and Energy: _____

_____

Post-Workout Food/Snack: _____

_____

_____

Notes: _____

_____

_____

_____

_____

| MUSCLE GROUP | SET 1 | | SET 2 | | SET 3 | | SET 4 | | SET 5 | |
| --- | --- | --- | --- | --- | --- | --- | --- | --- | --- | --- |
| EXERCISE | REPS | WGT | REPS | WGT | REPS | WGT | REPS | WGT | REPS | WGT |
| | | | | | | | | | | |
| | | | | | | | | | | |
| | | | | | | | | | | |
| | | | | | | | | | | |
| | | | | | | | | | | |
| | | | | | | | | | | |
| | | | | | | | | | | |
| | | | | | | | | | | |
| | | | | | | | | | | |
| | | | | | | | | | | |
| | | | | | | | | | | |
| | | | | | | | | | | |

Date: _____

Day of the Week: S ☐   M ☐   T ☐   W ☐   R ☐   F ☐   S ☐

Start Time: _____   Finish Time: _____

Stretch/Warm-Up: Yes ☐   No ☐

Cardio: _____   Level: _____

Pre-Workout Mood and Energy: _____

Pre-Workout Food/Snack: _____

## MUSCLE GROUP EMPHASIZED

Chest ☐   Shoulders ☐   Back ☐   Arms ☐
Legs ☐   Abs ☐   None ☐

## WORKOUT QUALITY

Low ☐   Okay ☐   Good ☐   Great ☐

Post-Workout Mood and Energy: _____

_____

Post-Workout Food/Snack: _____

_____

_____

Notes: _____

_____

_____

_____

_____

_____

| MUSCLE GROUP | SET 1 | | SET 2 | | SET 3 | | SET 4 | | SET 5 | |
| --- | --- | --- | --- | --- | --- | --- | --- | --- | --- | --- |
| EXERCISE | REPS | WGT | REPS | WGT | REPS | WGT | REPS | WGT | REPS | WGT |
| | | | | | | | | | | |
| | | | | | | | | | | |
| | | | | | | | | | | |
| | | | | | | | | | | |
| | | | | | | | | | | |
| | | | | | | | | | | |
| | | | | | | | | | | |
| | | | | | | | | | | |
| | | | | | | | | | | |
| | | | | | | | | | | |
| | | | | | | | | | | |
| | | | | | | | | | | |

Date: _____

Day of the Week:  S ☐     M ☐     T ☐     W ☐     R ☐     F ☐     S ☐

Start Time: _____     Finish Time: _____

Stretch/Warm-Up:  Yes ☐     No ☐

Cardio: _____     Level: _____

Pre-Workout Mood and Energy: _____

Pre-Workout Food/Snack: _____

## MUSCLE GROUP EMPHASIZED

Chest ☐     Shoulders ☐     Back ☐     Arms ☐
Legs ☐     Abs ☐     None ☐

## WORKOUT QUALITY

Low ☐     Okay ☐     Good ☐     Great ☐

Post-Workout Mood and Energy: _____

_____

Post-Workout Food/Snack: _____

_____

_____

Notes: _____

_____

_____

_____

_____

_____

| MUSCLE GROUP | SET 1 | | SET 2 | | SET 3 | | SET 4 | | SET 5 | |
|---|---|---|---|---|---|---|---|---|---|---|
| EXERCISE | REPS | WGT | REPS | WGT | REPS | WGT | REPS | WGT | REPS | WGT |
| | | | | | | | | | | |
| | | | | | | | | | | |
| | | | | | | | | | | |
| | | | | | | | | | | |
| | | | | | | | | | | |
| | | | | | | | | | | |
| | | | | | | | | | | |
| | | | | | | | | | | |
| | | | | | | | | | | |
| | | | | | | | | | | |
| | | | | | | | | | | |
| | | | | | | | | | | |

Date: _____

Day of the Week: S ☐  M ☐  T ☐  W ☐  R ☐  F ☐  S ☐

Start Time: _____  Finish Time: _____

Stretch/Warm-Up: Yes ☐  No ☐

Cardio: _____  Level: _____

Pre-Workout Mood and Energy: _____

Pre-Workout Food/Snack: _____

## MUSCLE GROUP EMPHASIZED

Chest ☐  Shoulders ☐  Back ☐  Arms ☐
Legs ☐  Abs ☐  None ☐

## WORKOUT QUALITY

Low ☐  Okay ☐  Good ☐  Great ☐

Post-Workout Mood and Energy: _____

_____

Post-Workout Food/Snack: _____

_____

_____

Notes: _____

_____

_____

_____

_____

_____

| MUSCLE GROUP | SET 1 | | SET 2 | | SET 3 | | SET 4 | | SET 5 | |
|---|---|---|---|---|---|---|---|---|---|---|
| EXERCISE | REPS | WGT | REPS | WGT | REPS | WGT | REPS | WGT | REPS | WGT |
| | | | | | | | | | | |
| | | | | | | | | | | |
| | | | | | | | | | | |
| | | | | | | | | | | |
| | | | | | | | | | | |
| | | | | | | | | | | |
| | | | | | | | | | | |
| | | | | | | | | | | |
| | | | | | | | | | | |
| | | | | | | | | | | |
| | | | | | | | | | | |
| | | | | | | | | | | |

Date: _____

Day of the Week:  S ☐    M ☐    T ☐    W ☐    R ☐    F ☐    S ☐

Start Time: _____    Finish Time: _____

Stretch/Warm-Up:  Yes ☐    No ☐

Cardio: _____    Level: _____

Pre-Workout Mood and Energy: _____

Pre-Workout Food/Snack: _____

## MUSCLE GROUP EMPHASIZED
Chest ☐    Shoulders ☐    Back ☐    Arms ☐
Legs ☐    Abs ☐    None ☐

## WORKOUT QUALITY
Low ☐    Okay ☐    Good ☐    Great ☐

Post-Workout Mood and Energy: _____

_____

Post-Workout Food/Snack: _____

_____

_____

Notes: _____

_____

_____

_____

_____

_____

| MUSCLE GROUP | SET 1 | | SET 2 | | SET 3 | | SET 4 | | SET 5 | |
|---|---|---|---|---|---|---|---|---|---|---|
| EXERCISE | REPS | WGT | REPS | WGT | REPS | WGT | REPS | WGT | REPS | WGT |
| | | | | | | | | | | |
| | | | | | | | | | | |
| | | | | | | | | | | |
| | | | | | | | | | | |
| | | | | | | | | | | |
| | | | | | | | | | | |
| | | | | | | | | | | |
| | | | | | | | | | | |
| | | | | | | | | | | |
| | | | | | | | | | | |
| | | | | | | | | | | |
| | | | | | | | | | | |
| | | | | | | | | | | |

Date: _____

Day of the Week:  S ☐    M ☐    T ☐    W ☐    R ☐    F ☐    S ☐

Start Time: _____    Finish Time: _____

Stretch/Warm-Up:  Yes ☐    No ☐

Cardio: _____    Level: _____

Pre-Workout Mood and Energy: _____

Pre-Workout Food/Snack: _____

## MUSCLE GROUP EMPHASIZED

Chest ☐    Shoulders ☐    Back ☐    Arms ☐
Legs ☐    Abs ☐    None ☐

## WORKOUT QUALITY

Low ☐    Okay ☐    Good ☐    Great ☐

Post-Workout Mood and Energy: _____

_____

Post-Workout Food/Snack: _____

_____

_____

Notes: _____

_____

_____

_____

_____

_____

| MUSCLE GROUP | SET 1 | | SET 2 | | SET 3 | | SET 4 | | SET 5 | |
|---|---|---|---|---|---|---|---|---|---|---|
| EXERCISE | REPS | WGT | REPS | WGT | REPS | WGT | REPS | WGT | REPS | WGT |
| | | | | | | | | | | |
| | | | | | | | | | | |
| | | | | | | | | | | |
| | | | | | | | | | | |
| | | | | | | | | | | |
| | | | | | | | | | | |
| | | | | | | | | | | |
| | | | | | | | | | | |
| | | | | | | | | | | |
| | | | | | | | | | | |
| | | | | | | | | | | |
| | | | | | | | | | | |

Date: _____

Day of the Week:  S ☐    M ☐    T ☐    W ☐    R ☐    F ☐    S ☐

Start Time: _____    Finish Time: _____

Stretch/Warm-Up:  Yes ☐    No ☐

Cardio: _____    Level: _____

Pre-Workout Mood and Energy: _____

Pre-Workout Food/Snack: _____

## MUSCLE GROUP EMPHASIZED

Chest ☐    Shoulders ☐    Back ☐    Arms ☐
Legs ☐    Abs ☐    None ☐

## WORKOUT QUALITY

Low ☐    Okay ☐    Good ☐    Great ☐

Post-Workout Mood and Energy: _____

_____

Post-Workout Food/Snack: _____

_____

_____

Notes: _____

_____

_____

_____

_____

_____

| MUSCLE GROUP | SET 1 | | SET 2 | | SET 3 | | SET 4 | | SET 5 | |
|---|---|---|---|---|---|---|---|---|---|---|
| EXERCISE | REPS | WGT | REPS | WGT | REPS | WGT | REPS | WGT | REPS | WGT |
| | | | | | | | | | | |
| | | | | | | | | | | |
| | | | | | | | | | | |
| | | | | | | | | | | |
| | | | | | | | | | | |
| | | | | | | | | | | |
| | | | | | | | | | | |
| | | | | | | | | | | |
| | | | | | | | | | | |
| | | | | | | | | | | |
| | | | | | | | | | | |

Date: _____

Day of the Week: S ☐   M ☐   T ☐   W ☐   R ☐   F ☐   S ☐

Start Time: _____   Finish Time: _____

Stretch/Warm-Up: Yes ☐   No ☐

Cardio: _____   Level: _____

Pre-Workout Mood and Energy: _____

Pre-Workout Food/Snack: _____

## MUSCLE GROUP EMPHASIZED

Chest ☐   Shoulders ☐   Back ☐   Arms ☐
Legs ☐   Abs ☐   None ☐

## WORKOUT QUALITY

Low ☐   Okay ☐   Good ☐   Great ☐

Post-Workout Mood and Energy: _____

_____

Post-Workout Food/Snack: _____

_____

_____

Notes: _____

_____

_____

_____

_____

_____

| MUSCLE GROUP | SET 1 | | SET 2 | | SET 3 | | SET 4 | | SET 5 | |
|---|---|---|---|---|---|---|---|---|---|---|
| EXERCISE | REPS | WGT | REPS | WGT | REPS | WGT | REPS | WGT | REPS | WGT |
| | | | | | | | | | | |
| | | | | | | | | | | |
| | | | | | | | | | | |
| | | | | | | | | | | |
| | | | | | | | | | | |
| | | | | | | | | | | |
| | | | | | | | | | | |
| | | | | | | | | | | |
| | | | | | | | | | | |
| | | | | | | | | | | |
| | | | | | | | | | | |
| | | | | | | | | | | |
| | | | | | | | | | | |

Date: _____

Day of the Week: S ☐    M ☐    T ☐    W ☐    R ☐    F ☐    S ☐

Start Time: _____    Finish Time: _____

Stretch/Warm-Up: Yes ☐    No ☐

Cardio: _____    Level: _____

Pre-Workout Mood and Energy: _____

Pre-Workout Food/Snack: _____

## MUSCLE GROUP EMPHASIZED
Chest ☐    Shoulders ☐    Back ☐    Arms ☐
Legs ☐    Abs ☐    None ☐

## WORKOUT QUALITY
Low ☐    Okay ☐    Good ☐    Great ☐

Post-Workout Mood and Energy: _____

_____

Post-Workout Food/Snack: _____

_____

_____

Notes: _____

_____

_____

_____

_____

_____

| MUSCLE GROUP | SET 1 | | SET 2 | | SET 3 | | SET 4 | | SET 5 | |
|---|---|---|---|---|---|---|---|---|---|---|
| EXERCISE | REPS | WGT | REPS | WGT | REPS | WGT | REPS | WGT | REPS | WGT |
| | | | | | | | | | | |
| | | | | | | | | | | |
| | | | | | | | | | | |
| | | | | | | | | | | |
| | | | | | | | | | | |
| | | | | | | | | | | |
| | | | | | | | | | | |
| | | | | | | | | | | |
| | | | | | | | | | | |
| | | | | | | | | | | |
| | | | | | | | | | | |
| | | | | | | | | | | |

Date: _____

Day of the Week: S ☐ M ☐ T ☐ W ☐ R ☐ F ☐ S ☐

Start Time: _____ Finish Time: _____

Stretch/Warm-Up: Yes ☐ No ☐

Cardio: _____ Level: _____

Pre-Workout Mood and Energy: _____

Pre-Workout Food/Snack: _____

## MUSCLE GROUP EMPHASIZED

Chest ☐ Shoulders ☐ Back ☐ Arms ☐
Legs ☐ Abs ☐ None ☐

## WORKOUT QUALITY

Low ☐ Okay ☐ Good ☐ Great ☐

Post-Workout Mood and Energy: _____

_____

Post-Workout Food/Snack: _____

_____

_____

Notes: _____

_____

_____

_____

_____

_____

| MUSCLE GROUP | SET 1 | | SET 2 | | SET 3 | | SET 4 | | SET 5 | |
|---|---|---|---|---|---|---|---|---|---|---|
| EXERCISE | REPS | WGT | REPS | WGT | REPS | WGT | REPS | WGT | REPS | WGT |
| | | | | | | | | | | |
| | | | | | | | | | | |
| | | | | | | | | | | |
| | | | | | | | | | | |
| | | | | | | | | | | |
| | | | | | | | | | | |
| | | | | | | | | | | |
| | | | | | | | | | | |
| | | | | | | | | | | |
| | | | | | | | | | | |
| | | | | | | | | | | |

Date: _____

Day of the Week: S ☐   M ☐   T ☐   W ☐   R ☐   F ☐   S ☐

Start Time: _____   Finish Time: _____

Stretch/Warm-Up: Yes ☐   No ☐

Cardio: _____   Level: _____

Pre-Workout Mood and Energy: _____

Pre-Workout Food/Snack: _____

## MUSCLE GROUP EMPHASIZED

Chest ☐   Shoulders ☐   Back ☐   Arms ☐
Legs ☐   Abs ☐   None ☐

## WORKOUT QUALITY

Low ☐   Okay ☐   Good ☐   Great ☐

Post-Workout Mood and Energy: _____

_____

Post-Workout Food/Snack: _____

_____

_____

Notes: _____

_____

_____

_____

_____

_____

| MUSCLE GROUP | SET 1 | | SET 2 | | SET 3 | | SET 4 | | SET 5 | |
|---|---|---|---|---|---|---|---|---|---|---|
| EXERCISE | REPS | WGT | REPS | WGT | REPS | WGT | REPS | WGT | REPS | WGT |
| | | | | | | | | | | |
| | | | | | | | | | | |
| | | | | | | | | | | |
| | | | | | | | | | | |
| | | | | | | | | | | |
| | | | | | | | | | | |
| | | | | | | | | | | |
| | | | | | | | | | | |
| | | | | | | | | | | |
| | | | | | | | | | | |
| | | | | | | | | | | |
| | | | | | | | | | | |
| | | | | | | | | | | |

Date: _____

Day of the Week:  S ☐    M ☐    T ☐    W ☐    R ☐    F ☐    S ☐

Start Time: _____    Finish Time: _____

Stretch/Warm-Up:  Yes ☐    No ☐

Cardio: _____    Level: _____

Pre-Workout Mood and Energy: _____

Pre-Workout Food/Snack: _____

## MUSCLE GROUP EMPHASIZED

Chest ☐    Shoulders ☐    Back ☐    Arms ☐
Legs ☐    Abs ☐    None ☐

## WORKOUT QUALITY

Low ☐    Okay ☐    Good ☐    Great ☐

Post-Workout Mood and Energy: _____

_____

Post-Workout Food/Snack: _____

_____

_____

Notes: _____

_____

_____

_____

_____

_____

| MUSCLE GROUP | SET 1 | | SET 2 | | SET 3 | | SET 4 | | SET 5 | |
|---|---|---|---|---|---|---|---|---|---|---|
| EXERCISE | REPS | WGT | REPS | WGT | REPS | WGT | REPS | WGT | REPS | WGT |
| | | | | | | | | | | |
| | | | | | | | | | | |
| | | | | | | | | | | |
| | | | | | | | | | | |
| | | | | | | | | | | |
| | | | | | | | | | | |
| | | | | | | | | | | |
| | | | | | | | | | | |
| | | | | | | | | | | |
| | | | | | | | | | | |
| | | | | | | | | | | |
| | | | | | | | | | | |

Date: _____

Day of the Week:  S ☐   M ☐   T ☐   W ☐   R ☐   F ☐   S ☐

Start Time: _____   Finish Time: _____

Stretch/Warm-Up: Yes ☐   No ☐

Cardio: _____   Level: _____

Pre-Workout Mood and Energy: _____

Pre-Workout Food/Snack: _____

## MUSCLE GROUP EMPHASIZED

Chest ☐   Shoulders ☐   Back ☐   Arms ☐
Legs ☐   Abs ☐   None ☐

## WORKOUT QUALITY

Low ☐   Okay ☐   Good ☐   Great ☐

Post-Workout Mood and Energy: _____

_____

Post-Workout Food/Snack: _____

_____

_____

Notes: _____

_____

_____

_____

_____

_____

| MUSCLE GROUP | SET 1 | | SET 2 | | SET 3 | | SET 4 | | SET 5 | |
|---|---|---|---|---|---|---|---|---|---|---|
| EXERCISE | REPS | WGT | REPS | WGT | REPS | WGT | REPS | WGT | REPS | WGT |
| | | | | | | | | | | |
| | | | | | | | | | | |
| | | | | | | | | | | |
| | | | | | | | | | | |
| | | | | | | | | | | |
| | | | | | | | | | | |
| | | | | | | | | | | |
| | | | | | | | | | | |
| | | | | | | | | | | |
| | | | | | | | | | | |
| | | | | | | | | | | |
| | | | | | | | | | | |

Date: _____

Day of the Week:  S ☐    M ☐    T ☐    W ☐    R ☐    F ☐    S ☐

Start Time: _____    Finish Time: _____

Stretch/Warm-Up:  Yes ☐    No ☐

Cardio: _____    Level: _____

Pre-Workout Mood and Energy: _____

Pre-Workout Food/Snack: _____

## MUSCLE GROUP EMPHASIZED

Chest ☐    Shoulders ☐    Back ☐    Arms ☐
Legs ☐    Abs ☐    None ☐

## WORKOUT QUALITY

Low ☐    Okay ☐    Good ☐    Great ☐

Post-Workout Mood and Energy: _____

_____

Post-Workout Food/Snack: _____

_____

_____

Notes: _____

_____

_____

_____

_____

_____

| MUSCLE GROUP | SET 1 | | SET 2 | | SET 3 | | SET 4 | | SET 5 | |
|---|---|---|---|---|---|---|---|---|---|---|
| EXERCISE | REPS | WGT | REPS | WGT | REPS | WGT | REPS | WGT | REPS | WGT |
| | | | | | | | | | | |
| | | | | | | | | | | |
| | | | | | | | | | | |
| | | | | | | | | | | |
| | | | | | | | | | | |
| | | | | | | | | | | |
| | | | | | | | | | | |
| | | | | | | | | | | |
| | | | | | | | | | | |
| | | | | | | | | | | |
| | | | | | | | | | | |
| | | | | | | | | | | |

Date: _____

Day of the Week:  S ☐    M ☐    T ☐    W ☐    R ☐    F ☐    S ☐

Start Time: _____    Finish Time: _____

Stretch/Warm-Up:  Yes ☐    No ☐

Cardio: _____    Level: _____

Pre-Workout Mood and Energy: _____

Pre-Workout Food/Snack: _____

## MUSCLE GROUP EMPHASIZED

Chest ☐    Shoulders ☐    Back ☐    Arms ☐
Legs ☐    Abs ☐    None ☐

## WORKOUT QUALITY

Low ☐    Okay ☐    Good ☐    Great ☐

Post-Workout Mood and Energy: _____

_____

Post-Workout Food/Snack: _____

_____

_____

Notes: _____

_____

_____

_____

_____

_____

| MUSCLE GROUP | SET 1 | | SET 2 | | SET 3 | | SET 4 | | SET 5 | |
|---|---|---|---|---|---|---|---|---|---|---|
| EXERCISE | REPS | WGT | REPS | WGT | REPS | WGT | REPS | WGT | REPS | WGT |
| | | | | | | | | | | |
| | | | | | | | | | | |
| | | | | | | | | | | |
| | | | | | | | | | | |
| | | | | | | | | | | |
| | | | | | | | | | | |
| | | | | | | | | | | |
| | | | | | | | | | | |
| | | | | | | | | | | |
| | | | | | | | | | | |
| | | | | | | | | | | |
| | | | | | | | | | | |

Date: _____

Day of the Week:  S ☐   M ☐   T ☐   W ☐   R ☐   F ☐   S ☐

Start Time: _____   Finish Time: _____

Stretch/Warm-Up: Yes ☐   No ☐

Cardio: _____   Level: _____

Pre-Workout Mood and Energy: _____

Pre-Workout Food/Snack: _____

## MUSCLE GROUP EMPHASIZED

Chest ☐   Shoulders ☐   Back ☐   Arms ☐
Legs ☐   Abs ☐   None ☐

## WORKOUT QUALITY

Low ☐   Okay ☐   Good ☐   Great ☐

Post-Workout Mood and Energy: _____

_____

Post-Workout Food/Snack: _____

_____

_____

Notes: _____

_____

_____

_____

_____

_____

| MUSCLE GROUP | SET 1 | | SET 2 | | SET 3 | | SET 4 | | SET 5 | |
|---|---|---|---|---|---|---|---|---|---|---|
| EXERCISE | REPS | WGT | REPS | WGT | REPS | WGT | REPS | WGT | REPS | WGT |
| | | | | | | | | | | |
| | | | | | | | | | | |
| | | | | | | | | | | |
| | | | | | | | | | | |
| | | | | | | | | | | |
| | | | | | | | | | | |
| | | | | | | | | | | |
| | | | | | | | | | | |
| | | | | | | | | | | |
| | | | | | | | | | | |
| | | | | | | | | | | |
| | | | | | | | | | | |

Date: _____

Day of the Week: S ☐   M ☐   T ☐   W ☐   R ☐   F ☐   S ☐

Start Time: _____    Finish Time: _____

Stretch/Warm-Up: Yes ☐   No ☐

Cardio: _____    Level: _____

Pre-Workout Mood and Energy: _____

Pre-Workout Food/Snack: _____

### MUSCLE GROUP EMPHASIZED

Chest ☐    Shoulders ☐    Back ☐    Arms ☐
Legs ☐    Abs ☐    None ☐

### WORKOUT QUALITY

Low ☐    Okay ☐    Good ☐    Great ☐

Post-Workout Mood and Energy: _____

_____

Post-Workout Food/Snack: _____

_____

_____

Notes: _____

_____

_____

_____

_____

_____

| MUSCLE GROUP | SET 1 | | SET 2 | | SET 3 | | SET 4 | | SET 5 | |
| --- | --- | --- | --- | --- | --- | --- | --- | --- | --- | --- |
| EXERCISE | REPS | WGT | REPS | WGT | REPS | WGT | REPS | WGT | REPS | WGT |
| | | | | | | | | | | |
| | | | | | | | | | | |
| | | | | | | | | | | |
| | | | | | | | | | | |
| | | | | | | | | | | |
| | | | | | | | | | | |
| | | | | | | | | | | |
| | | | | | | | | | | |
| | | | | | | | | | | |
| | | | | | | | | | | |
| | | | | | | | | | | |
| | | | | | | | | | | |

Date: _____

Day of the Week:  S ☐    M ☐    T ☐    W ☐    R ☐    F ☐    S ☐

Start Time: _____    Finish Time: _____

Stretch/Warm-Up:  Yes ☐    No ☐

Cardio: _____    Level: _____

Pre-Workout Mood and Energy: _____

Pre-Workout Food/Snack: _____

## MUSCLE GROUP EMPHASIZED

Chest ☐    Shoulders ☐    Back ☐    Arms ☐
Legs ☐    Abs ☐    None ☐

## WORKOUT QUALITY

Low ☐    Okay ☐    Good ☐    Great ☐

Post-Workout Mood and Energy: _____

_____

Post-Workout Food/Snack: _____

_____

_____

Notes: _____

_____

_____

_____

_____

_____

| MUSCLE GROUP | SET 1 | | SET 2 | | SET 3 | | SET 4 | | SET 5 | |
|---|---|---|---|---|---|---|---|---|---|---|
| EXERCISE | REPS | WGT | REPS | WGT | REPS | WGT | REPS | WGT | REPS | WGT |
| | | | | | | | | | | |
| | | | | | | | | | | |
| | | | | | | | | | | |
| | | | | | | | | | | |
| | | | | | | | | | | |
| | | | | | | | | | | |
| | | | | | | | | | | |
| | | | | | | | | | | |
| | | | | | | | | | | |
| | | | | | | | | | | |
| | | | | | | | | | | |
| | | | | | | | | | | |

Date: _____

Day of the Week:  S ☐    M ☐    T ☐    W ☐    R ☐    F ☐    S ☐

Start Time: _____    Finish Time: _____

Stretch/Warm-Up:  Yes ☐    No ☐

Cardio: _____    Level: _____

Pre-Workout Mood and Energy: _____

Pre-Workout Food/Snack: _____

## MUSCLE GROUP EMPHASIZED

Chest ☐    Shoulders ☐    Back ☐    Arms ☐
Legs ☐    Abs ☐    None ☐

## WORKOUT QUALITY

Low ☐    Okay ☐    Good ☐    Great ☐

Post-Workout Mood and Energy: _____

_____

Post-Workout Food/Snack: _____

_____

_____

Notes: _____

_____

_____

_____

_____

_____

| MUSCLE GROUP | SET 1 | | SET 2 | | SET 3 | | SET 4 | | SET 5 | |
|---|---|---|---|---|---|---|---|---|---|---|
| EXERCISE | REPS | WGT | REPS | WGT | REPS | WGT | REPS | WGT | REPS | WGT |
| | | | | | | | | | | |
| | | | | | | | | | | |
| | | | | | | | | | | |
| | | | | | | | | | | |
| | | | | | | | | | | |
| | | | | | | | | | | |
| | | | | | | | | | | |
| | | | | | | | | | | |
| | | | | | | | | | | |
| | | | | | | | | | | |
| | | | | | | | | | | |

Date: _____

Day of the Week:  S ☐    M ☐    T ☐    W ☐    R ☐    F ☐    S ☐

Start Time: _____    Finish Time: _____

Stretch/Warm-Up:  Yes ☐    No ☐

Cardio: _____    Level: _____

Pre-Workout Mood and Energy: _____

Pre-Workout Food/Snack: _____

## MUSCLE GROUP EMPHASIZED

Chest ☐    Shoulders ☐    Back ☐    Arms ☐
Legs ☐    Abs ☐    None ☐

## WORKOUT QUALITY

Low ☐    Okay ☐    Good ☐    Great ☐

Post-Workout Mood and Energy: _____

_____

Post-Workout Food/Snack: _____

_____

_____

Notes: _____

_____

_____

_____

_____

_____

| MUSCLE GROUP | SET 1 | | SET 2 | | SET 3 | | SET 4 | | SET 5 | |
|---|---|---|---|---|---|---|---|---|---|---|
| EXERCISE | REPS | WGT | REPS | WGT | REPS | WGT | REPS | WGT | REPS | WGT |
| | | | | | | | | | | |
| | | | | | | | | | | |
| | | | | | | | | | | |
| | | | | | | | | | | |
| | | | | | | | | | | |
| | | | | | | | | | | |
| | | | | | | | | | | |
| | | | | | | | | | | |
| | | | | | | | | | | |
| | | | | | | | | | | |
| | | | | | | | | | | |
| | | | | | | | | | | |

Date: _____

Day of the Week:  S ☐    M ☐    T ☐    W ☐    R ☐    F ☐    S ☐

Start Time: _____    Finish Time: _____

Stretch/Warm-Up:  Yes ☐    No ☐

Cardio: _____    Level: _____

Pre-Workout Mood and Energy: _____

Pre-Workout Food/Snack: _____

## MUSCLE GROUP EMPHASIZED

Chest ☐    Shoulders ☐    Back ☐    Arms ☐
Legs ☐    Abs ☐    None ☐

## WORKOUT QUALITY

Low ☐    Okay ☐    Good ☐    Great ☐

Post-Workout Mood and Energy: _____

_____

Post-Workout Food/Snack: _____

_____

_____

Notes: _____

_____

_____

_____

_____

_____

| MUSCLE GROUP | SET 1 | | SET 2 | | SET 3 | | SET 4 | | SET 5 | |
|---|---|---|---|---|---|---|---|---|---|---|
| EXERCISE | REPS | WGT | REPS | WGT | REPS | WGT | REPS | WGT | REPS | WGT |
| | | | | | | | | | | |
| | | | | | | | | | | |
| | | | | | | | | | | |
| | | | | | | | | | | |
| | | | | | | | | | | |
| | | | | | | | | | | |
| | | | | | | | | | | |
| | | | | | | | | | | |
| | | | | | | | | | | |
| | | | | | | | | | | |
| | | | | | | | | | | |

Date: _____

Day of the Week:  S ☐    M ☐    T ☐    W ☐    R ☐    F ☐    S ☐

Start Time: _____    Finish Time: _____

Stretch/Warm-Up:  Yes ☐    No ☐

Cardio: _____    Level: _____

Pre-Workout Mood and Energy: _____

Pre-Workout Food/Snack: _____

## MUSCLE GROUP EMPHASIZED

Chest ☐    Shoulders ☐    Back ☐    Arms ☐
Legs ☐    Abs ☐    None ☐

## WORKOUT QUALITY

Low ☐    Okay ☐    Good ☐    Great ☐

Post-Workout Mood and Energy: _____

_____

Post-Workout Food/Snack: _____

_____

_____

Notes: _____

_____

_____

_____

_____

_____

| MUSCLE GROUP | SET 1 | | SET 2 | | SET 3 | | SET 4 | | SET 5 | |
|---|---|---|---|---|---|---|---|---|---|---|
| EXERCISE | REPS | WGT | REPS | WGT | REPS | WGT | REPS | WGT | REPS | WGT |
| | | | | | | | | | | |
| | | | | | | | | | | |
| | | | | | | | | | | |
| | | | | | | | | | | |
| | | | | | | | | | | |
| | | | | | | | | | | |
| | | | | | | | | | | |
| | | | | | | | | | | |
| | | | | | | | | | | |
| | | | | | | | | | | |

Date: _____

Day of the Week:  S ☐    M ☐    T ☐    W ☐    R ☐    F ☐    S ☐

Start Time: _____    Finish Time: _____

Stretch/Warm-Up:  Yes ☐    No ☐

Cardio: _____    Level: _____

Pre-Workout Mood and Energy: _____

Pre-Workout Food/Snack: _____

## MUSCLE GROUP EMPHASIZED

Chest ☐    Shoulders ☐    Back ☐    Arms ☐
Legs ☐    Abs ☐    None ☐

## WORKOUT QUALITY

Low ☐    Okay ☐    Good ☐    Great ☐

Post-Workout Mood and Energy: _____

_____

Post-Workout Food/Snack: _____

_____

_____

Notes: _____

_____

_____

_____

_____

_____

| MUSCLE GROUP | SET 1 | | SET 2 | | SET 3 | | SET 4 | | SET 5 | |
|---|---|---|---|---|---|---|---|---|---|---|
| EXERCISE | REPS | WGT | REPS | WGT | REPS | WGT | REPS | WGT | REPS | WGT |
| | | | | | | | | | | |
| | | | | | | | | | | |
| | | | | | | | | | | |
| | | | | | | | | | | |
| | | | | | | | | | | |
| | | | | | | | | | | |
| | | | | | | | | | | |
| | | | | | | | | | | |
| | | | | | | | | | | |
| | | | | | | | | | | |
| | | | | | | | | | | |

Date: _____

Day of the Week:  S ☐    M ☐    T ☐    W ☐    R ☐    F ☐    S ☐

Start Time: _____    Finish Time: _____

Stretch/Warm-Up:  Yes ☐    No ☐

Cardio: _____    Level: _____

Pre-Workout Mood and Energy: _____

Pre-Workout Food/Snack: _____

### MUSCLE GROUP EMPHASIZED

Chest ☐    Shoulders ☐    Back ☐    Arms ☐
Legs ☐    Abs ☐    None ☐

### WORKOUT QUALITY

Low ☐    Okay ☐    Good ☐    Great ☐

Post-Workout Mood and Energy: _____

_____

Post-Workout Food/Snack: _____

_____

_____

Notes: _____

_____

_____

_____

_____

_____

| MUSCLE GROUP | SET 1 | | SET 2 | | SET 3 | | SET 4 | | SET 5 | |
|---|---|---|---|---|---|---|---|---|---|---|
| EXERCISE | REPS | WGT | REPS | WGT | REPS | WGT | REPS | WGT | REPS | WGT |
| | | | | | | | | | | |
| | | | | | | | | | | |
| | | | | | | | | | | |
| | | | | | | | | | | |
| | | | | | | | | | | |
| | | | | | | | | | | |
| | | | | | | | | | | |
| | | | | | | | | | | |
| | | | | | | | | | | |
| | | | | | | | | | | |
| | | | | | | | | | | |

Date: _____

Day of the Week:  S ☐   M ☐   T ☐   W ☐   R ☐   F ☐   S ☐

Start Time: _____    Finish Time: _____

Stretch/Warm-Up:  Yes ☐    No ☐

Cardio: _____    Level: _____

Pre-Workout Mood and Energy: _____

Pre-Workout Food/Snack: _____

## MUSCLE GROUP EMPHASIZED
Chest ☐    Shoulders ☐    Back ☐    Arms ☐
Legs ☐    Abs ☐    None ☐

## WORKOUT QUALITY
Low ☐    Okay ☐    Good ☐    Great ☐

Post-Workout Mood and Energy: _____

_____

Post-Workout Food/Snack: _____

_____

_____

Notes: _____

_____

_____

_____

_____

_____

| MUSCLE GROUP | SET 1 | | SET 2 | | SET 3 | | SET 4 | | SET 5 | |
|---|---|---|---|---|---|---|---|---|---|---|
| EXERCISE | REPS | WGT | REPS | WGT | REPS | WGT | REPS | WGT | REPS | WGT |
| | | | | | | | | | | |
| | | | | | | | | | | |
| | | | | | | | | | | |
| | | | | | | | | | | |
| | | | | | | | | | | |
| | | | | | | | | | | |
| | | | | | | | | | | |
| | | | | | | | | | | |
| | | | | | | | | | | |
| | | | | | | | | | | |
| | | | | | | | | | | |
| | | | | | | | | | | |

Date: _____

Day of the Week:  S ☐     M ☐     T ☐     W ☐     R ☐     F ☐     S ☐

Start Time: _____     Finish Time: _____

Stretch/Warm-Up:  Yes ☐     No ☐

Cardio: _____     Level: _____

Pre-Workout Mood and Energy: _____

Pre-Workout Food/Snack: _____

## MUSCLE GROUP EMPHASIZED

Chest ☐     Shoulders ☐     Back ☐     Arms ☐
Legs ☐     Abs ☐     None ☐

## WORKOUT QUALITY

Low ☐     Okay ☐     Good ☐     Great ☐

Post-Workout Mood and Energy: _____

_____

Post-Workout Food/Snack: _____

_____

_____

Notes: _____

_____

_____

_____

_____

_____

| MUSCLE GROUP | SET 1 | | SET 2 | | SET 3 | | SET 4 | | SET 5 | |
|---|---|---|---|---|---|---|---|---|---|---|
| **EXERCISE** | REPS | WGT | REPS | WGT | REPS | WGT | REPS | WGT | REPS | WGT |
| | | | | | | | | | | |
| | | | | | | | | | | |
| | | | | | | | | | | |
| | | | | | | | | | | |
| | | | | | | | | | | |
| | | | | | | | | | | |
| | | | | | | | | | | |
| | | | | | | | | | | |
| | | | | | | | | | | |
| | | | | | | | | | | |
| | | | | | | | | | | |

Date: _____

Day of the Week: S ☐   M ☐   T ☐   W ☐   R ☐   F ☐   S ☐

Start Time: _____   Finish Time: _____

Stretch/Warm-Up: Yes ☐   No ☐

Cardio: _____   Level: _____

Pre-Workout Mood and Energy: _____

Pre-Workout Food/Snack: _____

## MUSCLE GROUP EMPHASIZED

Chest ☐   Shoulders ☐   Back ☐   Arms ☐
Legs ☐   Abs ☐   None ☐

## WORKOUT QUALITY

Low ☐   Okay ☐   Good ☐   Great ☐

Post-Workout Mood and Energy: _____

_____

Post-Workout Food/Snack: _____

_____

_____

Notes: _____

_____

_____

_____

_____

| MUSCLE GROUP | SET 1 | | SET 2 | | SET 3 | | SET 4 | | SET 5 | |
|---|---|---|---|---|---|---|---|---|---|---|
| EXERCISE | REPS | WGT | REPS | WGT | REPS | WGT | REPS | WGT | REPS | WGT |
| | | | | | | | | | | |
| | | | | | | | | | | |
| | | | | | | | | | | |
| | | | | | | | | | | |
| | | | | | | | | | | |
| | | | | | | | | | | |
| | | | | | | | | | | |
| | | | | | | | | | | |
| | | | | | | | | | | |
| | | | | | | | | | | |
| | | | | | | | | | | |
| | | | | | | | | | | |

Date: _____

Day of the Week:  S ☐    M ☐    T ☐    W ☐    R ☐    F ☐    S ☐

Start Time: _____    Finish Time: _____

Stretch/Warm-Up:  Yes ☐    No ☐

Cardio: _____    Level: _____

Pre-Workout Mood and Energy: _____

Pre-Workout Food/Snack: _____

## MUSCLE GROUP EMPHASIZED

Chest ☐    Shoulders ☐    Back ☐    Arms ☐
Legs ☐    Abs ☐    None ☐

## WORKOUT QUALITY

Low ☐    Okay ☐    Good ☐    Great ☐

Post-Workout Mood and Energy: _____

_____

Post-Workout Food/Snack: _____

_____

_____

Notes: _____

_____

_____

_____

_____

_____

| MUSCLE GROUP | SET 1 | | SET 2 | | SET 3 | | SET 4 | | SET 5 | |
|---|---|---|---|---|---|---|---|---|---|---|
| EXERCISE | REPS | WGT | REPS | WGT | REPS | WGT | REPS | WGT | REPS | WGT |
| | | | | | | | | | | |
| | | | | | | | | | | |
| | | | | | | | | | | |
| | | | | | | | | | | |
| | | | | | | | | | | |
| | | | | | | | | | | |
| | | | | | | | | | | |
| | | | | | | | | | | |
| | | | | | | | | | | |
| | | | | | | | | | | |
| | | | | | | | | | | |
| | | | | | | | | | | |

Date: _____

Day of the Week:  S ☐    M ☐    T ☐    W ☐    R ☐    F ☐    S ☐

Start Time: _____    Finish Time: _____

Stretch/Warm-Up:  Yes ☐    No ☐

Cardio: _____    Level: _____

Pre-Workout Mood and Energy: _____

Pre-Workout Food/Snack: _____

## MUSCLE GROUP EMPHASIZED

Chest ☐     Shoulders ☐     Back ☐     Arms ☐
Legs ☐     Abs ☐     None ☐

## WORKOUT QUALITY

Low ☐     Okay ☐     Good ☐     Great ☐

Post-Workout Mood and Energy: _____

_____

Post-Workout Food/Snack: _____

_____

_____

Notes: _____

_____

_____

_____

_____

_____

| MUSCLE GROUP | SET 1 | | SET 2 | | SET 3 | | SET 4 | | SET 5 | |
|---|---|---|---|---|---|---|---|---|---|---|
| EXERCISE | REPS | WGT | REPS | WGT | REPS | WGT | REPS | WGT | REPS | WGT |
| | | | | | | | | | | |
| | | | | | | | | | | |
| | | | | | | | | | | |
| | | | | | | | | | | |
| | | | | | | | | | | |
| | | | | | | | | | | |
| | | | | | | | | | | |
| | | | | | | | | | | |
| | | | | | | | | | | |
| | | | | | | | | | | |
| | | | | | | | | | | |
| | | | | | | | | | | |

Date: _____

Day of the Week: S ☐   M ☐   T ☐   W ☐   R ☐   F ☐   S ☐

Start Time: _____   Finish Time: _____

Stretch/Warm-Up: Yes ☐   No ☐

Cardio: _____   Level: _____

Pre-Workout Mood and Energy: _____

Pre-Workout Food/Snack: _____

## MUSCLE GROUP EMPHASIZED
Chest ☐   Shoulders ☐   Back ☐   Arms ☐
Legs ☐   Abs ☐   None ☐

## WORKOUT QUALITY
Low ☐   Okay ☐   Good ☐   Great ☐

Post-Workout Mood and Energy: _____

_____

Post-Workout Food/Snack: _____

_____

_____

Notes: _____

_____

_____

_____

_____

_____

| MUSCLE GROUP | SET 1 | | SET 2 | | SET 3 | | SET 4 | | SET 5 | |
|---|---|---|---|---|---|---|---|---|---|---|
| EXERCISE | REPS | WGT | REPS | WGT | REPS | WGT | REPS | WGT | REPS | WGT |
| | | | | | | | | | | |
| | | | | | | | | | | |
| | | | | | | | | | | |
| | | | | | | | | | | |
| | | | | | | | | | | |
| | | | | | | | | | | |
| | | | | | | | | | | |
| | | | | | | | | | | |
| | | | | | | | | | | |
| | | | | | | | | | | |
| | | | | | | | | | | |
| | | | | | | | | | | |

Date: _____

Day of the Week: S ☐    M ☐    T ☐    W ☐    R ☐    F ☐    S ☐

Start Time: _____    Finish Time: _____

Stretch/Warm-Up: Yes ☐    No ☐

Cardio: _____    Level: _____

Pre-Workout Mood and Energy: _____

Pre-Workout Food/Snack: _____

## MUSCLE GROUP EMPHASIZED

Chest ☐    Shoulders ☐    Back ☐    Arms ☐
Legs ☐    Abs ☐    None ☐

## WORKOUT QUALITY

Low ☐    Okay ☐    Good ☐    Great ☐

Post-Workout Mood and Energy: _____

_____

Post-Workout Food/Snack: _____

_____

_____

Notes: _____

_____

_____

_____

_____

_____

| MUSCLE GROUP | SET 1 | | SET 2 | | SET 3 | | SET 4 | | SET 5 | |
|---|---|---|---|---|---|---|---|---|---|---|
| EXERCISE | REPS | WGT | REPS | WGT | REPS | WGT | REPS | WGT | REPS | WGT |
| | | | | | | | | | | |
| | | | | | | | | | | |
| | | | | | | | | | | |
| | | | | | | | | | | |
| | | | | | | | | | | |
| | | | | | | | | | | |
| | | | | | | | | | | |
| | | | | | | | | | | |
| | | | | | | | | | | |
| | | | | | | | | | | |
| | | | | | | | | | | |
| | | | | | | | | | | |

Date: _____

Day of the Week: S ☐   M ☐   T ☐   W ☐   R ☐   F ☐   S ☐

Start Time: _____   Finish Time: _____

Stretch/Warm-Up: Yes ☐   No ☐

Cardio: _____   Level: _____

Pre-Workout Mood and Energy: _____

Pre-Workout Food/Snack: _____

## MUSCLE GROUP EMPHASIZED

Chest ☐   Shoulders ☐   Back ☐   Arms ☐
Legs ☐   Abs ☐   None ☐

## WORKOUT QUALITY

Low ☐   Okay ☐   Good ☐   Great ☐

Post-Workout Mood and Energy: _____

_____

Post-Workout Food/Snack: _____

_____

_____

Notes: _____

_____

_____

_____

_____

_____

| MUSCLE GROUP | SET 1 | | SET 2 | | SET 3 | | SET 4 | | SET 5 | |
|---|---|---|---|---|---|---|---|---|---|---|
| EXERCISE | REPS | WGT | REPS | WGT | REPS | WGT | REPS | WGT | REPS | WGT |
| | | | | | | | | | | |
| | | | | | | | | | | |
| | | | | | | | | | | |
| | | | | | | | | | | |
| | | | | | | | | | | |
| | | | | | | | | | | |
| | | | | | | | | | | |
| | | | | | | | | | | |
| | | | | | | | | | | |
| | | | | | | | | | | |
| | | | | | | | | | | |
| | | | | | | | | | | |

Date: _____

Day of the Week: S ☐   M ☐   T ☐   W ☐   R ☐   F ☐   S ☐

Start Time: _____   Finish Time: _____

Stretch/Warm-Up: Yes ☐   No ☐

Cardio: _____   Level: _____

Pre-Workout Mood and Energy: _____

Pre-Workout Food/Snack: _____

## MUSCLE GROUP EMPHASIZED

Chest ☐   Shoulders ☐   Back ☐   Arms ☐
Legs ☐   Abs ☐   None ☐

## WORKOUT QUALITY

Low ☐   Okay ☐   Good ☐   Great ☐

Post-Workout Mood and Energy: _____

_____

Post-Workout Food/Snack: _____

_____

_____

Notes: _____

_____

_____

_____

_____

_____

| MUSCLE GROUP | SET 1 | | SET 2 | | SET 3 | | SET 4 | | SET 5 | |
|---|---|---|---|---|---|---|---|---|---|---|
| EXERCISE | REPS | WGT | REPS | WGT | REPS | WGT | REPS | WGT | REPS | WGT |
| | | | | | | | | | | |
| | | | | | | | | | | |
| | | | | | | | | | | |
| | | | | | | | | | | |
| | | | | | | | | | | |
| | | | | | | | | | | |
| | | | | | | | | | | |
| | | | | | | | | | | |
| | | | | | | | | | | |
| | | | | | | | | | | |
| | | | | | | | | | | |

Date: _____

Day of the Week:  S ☐   M ☐   T ☐   W ☐   R ☐   F ☐   S ☐

Start Time: _____    Finish Time: _____

Stretch/Warm-Up:  Yes ☐    No ☐

Cardio: _____    Level: _____

Pre-Workout Mood and Energy: _____

Pre-Workout Food/Snack: _____

## MUSCLE GROUP EMPHASIZED

Chest ☐    Shoulders ☐    Back ☐    Arms ☐
Legs ☐    Abs ☐    None ☐

## WORKOUT QUALITY

Low ☐    Okay ☐    Good ☐    Great ☐

Post-Workout Mood and Energy: _____

_____

Post-Workout Food/Snack: _____

_____

_____

Notes: _____

_____

_____

_____

_____

_____

| MUSCLE GROUP | SET 1 | | SET 2 | | SET 3 | | SET 4 | | SET 5 | |
|---|---|---|---|---|---|---|---|---|---|---|
| EXERCISE | REPS | WGT | REPS | WGT | REPS | WGT | REPS | WGT | REPS | WGT |
| | | | | | | | | | | |
| | | | | | | | | | | |
| | | | | | | | | | | |
| | | | | | | | | | | |
| | | | | | | | | | | |
| | | | | | | | | | | |
| | | | | | | | | | | |
| | | | | | | | | | | |
| | | | | | | | | | | |
| | | | | | | | | | | |
| | | | | | | | | | | |
| | | | | | | | | | | |

# EXERCISES BY BODY PART

## CHEST

Push-Ups (regular, incline, or decline)

Fat Barbell or Dumbbell Bench Press

Incline Barbell or Dumbbell Bench Press

Decline Barbell or Dumbbell Bench Press

Chest Press Machine

Peck Deck Machine

Bodyweight or Weighted Dips

Cable Crossovers or Chest Fly

## BICEPS

Standing Barbell, Dumbbell, or EZ Bar Curls

Standing or Seated Dumbbell Hammer Curls or Cross-Body Curls

Barbell, Dumbbell, or EZ Bar Preacher Curls

Seated Dumbbell Curls or Seated Incline Dumbbells Curls

Concentration Curls with Dumbbell or Cable

Cable Curls or Cable Hammer Curls

Bicep Curl Machine or Preacher Curl Machine

## TRICEPS

Bodyweight or Weighted Dips on Bench or Bars

Narrow Grip Push-Up

Close-Grip Bench Press or Dumbbell Press

Seated or Standing Tricep Extension with Cables, Dumbbells, or Barbell

Skull Crushers with Dumbbells or Barbell

Tricep Kickbacks with Dumbbells or Cables

## BACK

Bodyweight, Assisted, or Banded Pull-Ups

Machine Lat Pull-Downs

Bent-Over Barbell or Smith Machine Rows

Single-Arm Dumbbell or Cable Rows

T-Bar or Landmine Rows

Seated Machine Rows

Chest-Supported Row with Dumbbells, Barbell, or Cables

Shrugs with Machine or Dumbbells

## SHOULDERS

Standing Overhead Press with Barbell or Dumbbells

Seated Overhead Press with Barbell or Dumbbells

Seated or Standing Machine Press or Smith Machine Press

Standing Upright Row with Dumbbells, Smith Machine, or Barbells

Seated or Standing Lateral Raise with Dumbbells or Cables

Seated or Standing Front Raise with Dumbbells, Barbell, Plate, or Cables

Seated or Standing Rear Delt Fly with Dumbbells, Plate, or Cables

Arnold Press

## QUADS

Rear Barbell or Dumbbell Squats

Front Barbell or Dumbbell Squats

Bulgarian Split Squats with Dumbbells or Barbell

Walking Lunges with Barbell or Dumbbells

Smith Machine Squat or Lunge

Leg Press

Dumbbell or Barbell Step-Up

Leg Extension

Machine Squat or Hack Squat

Sissy Squat

## HAMSTRINGS

Straight Leg Deadlifts with Barbell, Smith Machine, or Dumbbells

Traditional Deadlift with Barbell, Smith Machine, or Dumbbells

Barbell or Dumbbell Sumo Deadlift

Lying or Seated Leg Curls

Single-Leg Dumbbell or Kettlebell Deadlift

## GLUTES

Hip Thrust with Barbell or Dumbbell

Good Morning with Barbell or Smith Machine

Cable Pull-Throughs

Hyperextensions

Glute-Ham Raises

Kickbacks with Cable or Machine

Abductor Machine

## ABS

Russian Twist

Dumbbell Crunch

Dumbbell Crossover Punch

Jackknife Pullover

Hanging Leg Raise

Planks

# RESOURCES

Check out these additional tools and learning guides to support your efforts to build a strong, healthy body:

Proper nutrition is key, and you can find your proper caloric intake by using an online calculator. I recommend **Leigh Peele's calculator** that can be found here: LeighPeele.com/mifflin-st-jeor-calculator.

Not sure how much of what to eat? A macro-tracking app is a great place to start. I recommend trying out the **MyFitnessPal** app. A browser version can be found here: MyFitnessPal.com.

Supplements are a great way to support a consistent nutrition and training plan. **BodyBuilding.com** has a great beginners guide on supplements, which can be found here: BodyBuilding.com/content/beginners-supplement-guide-5-supplements-you-need-now.html.

Unsure where to begin when it comes to your workouts? **MuscleandStrength.com** has several workout routines for you to try. They can be found here: MuscleandStrength.com/workout-routines.

Don't forget to make time for recovery! Yoga is a great option for mobility, flexibility, and strength. The YouTube channel, **Yoga With Adriene**, provides tons of great, high-quality free yoga videos. Her channel can be found here: YouTube.com/user/yogawithadriene.

# ABOUT THE AUTHOR

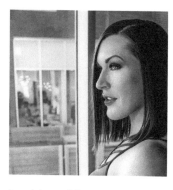

**KALLI YOUNGSTROM** is a health and wellness entrepreneur from Saskatoon, Saskatchewan, who uses her experiences as a lifelong athlete, professional body builder and world-level powerlifter to guide others in living their healthiest, happiest, and strongest lives. With nearly a decade of experience in health and fitness coaching, Kalli works with both women and men internationally. She has aided thousands in increasing their quality of life through physical fitness and nutrition coaching, with an emphasis on mental and emotional health. Kalli holds degrees in psychology and marketing as well as certificates in personal training, weight management, mindful meditation, and sports and personal nutrition. She works to bridge the gap between the mind and body in order to guide others in becoming the best version of themselves, and to provide them with tools and resources to do so. Find Kalli on Instagram at @kalliyoungstrom and at her website KYFitness.ca, or send her an email at kyfitnessandnutrition@gmail.com to learn more.